OVERCOME DIABETES

STOP MAKING EXCUSES
RESIST THE HYPE
SAVE YOUR LIFE

MARIAN HAYS

Books may be purchased in quantity by contacting the publisher at Info@CSPress.io or by calling 972-377-0607.

Book Consultant: Judith Briles, The Book Shepherd, TheBookShepherd.com
Front Cover Graphic: Nick Zelinger, NZGraphics.com
Cover design, interior design, and eBook conversion:
Rebecca Finkel, F+P Graphic Design, FPGD.com

ISBN paper: 978-0-9984369-5-1
ISBN eBook 978-0-9984369-3-7
ISBN audiobook 978-0-9984369-4-4

HEALTH | NUTRITION | DIABETES

Praise for *Overcome Diabetes*

Back home in Mexico my family always talk about diabetes and what's going to happen to their health, but no one ever said what to do to prevent it or how to help someone with diabetes. I don't have diabetes, but I have relatives and friends with diabetes. This information will help me gain insight into their challenges and bring them solutions. I recommend this book!

—ANAYELI BENITEZ, Wife, mom, marathon runner

Coming from a long line of type 2 diabetics, myself included, the possibility of improving instead of steadily progressing with more and more meds is certainly something that many of us would be happy to know more about.

—CAROL BREMNER, Type 2 Diabetic, Internet trainer and consultant

Great Resource for Diabetics and Family Members! A great resource for anyone who wants to know more about their diet options as a diabetic, or anyone who has a diabetic family member and needs to know better how to prepare meals and plan what foods to serve. There is a lot of important information in this book that no diabetic should be without.

—JOANNA MARTIN, Diabetic family member

While I don't have diabetes, I keep hearing of others who do. I thought it would be good to have a book to refer folks to—which I did immediately upon finishing reading it. I suggested my library get a copy, which they did.

—CYNTHIA ANN LEIGHTON, Owner, Software Enterprise Limited

Other Books by Marian Hays

Diabetes Diet Options

Diabetes Journal

Healthy Brain, Better Life

Eating Smarter, Living Better Journal

Low-Carb Recipes and Journal

Low-Calorie Recipes and Journal

Contents

1
PART

1

Why This Book?

Let us first understand the facts,
and then we may seek the cause.
—ARISTOTLE

After I wrote *Diabetes Diet Options,* I noticed how many people knew they should take better care of themselves, exercise, change their diet, and track results. But they didn't.

I see people who want to reverse their diabetes or prevent their prediabetes from progressing to a type 2 diagnosis. But they're struggling. What they've tried hasn't worked. They are expecting or hoping the drugs will do the job for them but hate taking the drugs at the same time. Many ignore the consequences because they don't really understand what they are or what, if anything, can be done about it.

Many simply ignore it because they can't imagine it happening to them. They don't know or understand the connection between what they do today affecting a diagnosis years later.

I've encouraged many friends and clients about how to have a healthy lifestyle. Some were happy to get the information, and others were simply discouraged or in denial.

An unexpected discovery came from a book about anti-aging, *Change Your Brain, Change Your Age* by Dr. Daniel Amen. I started reading it from the anti-aging perspective and quickly realized how much we can change our diabetes issues by understanding how to have a healthy brain.

Dr. Amen has written several brain health books, and they all share fascinating stories and information about how our brains work, what they need for optimal health, and what compromises our health, resulting in unnecessary disease. And disease leads to faster aging. The most powerful fact is that we can heal our brains, reverse disease, and extend our lives.

I was on a new quest. I dug into multiple resources and got a much bigger picture of what affects our behavior, habits, and ability to make the changes we want to make. Our wonderfully created bodies are an intricate system knit together with billions of cells and elaborate connections.

I saw how many of us have come to believe diabetic myths that get passed on as facts. When you believe them, you probably won't work very hard to overcome them, feeling instead like you're stuck with a sad life sentence and thus make excuses for not changing.

It's not all excuses and myths, though. We're confronted with an incredible amount of hype and sabotage. This means we have internal and external influences that affect our progress in overcoming diabetes.

The more I read, the more I felt pulled to write this book about overcoming the challenges that stop us from restoring our health.

There are over 20,000 books on Amazon alone that mention diabetes. They cover what it is, what to eat or not eat, menus, stories about people who have diabetes, and how it can be reversed. I didn't find any that focused specifically on how and why diabetics get stuck and what to do about it.

No one needs the doom and gloom dished out from the traditionally trained medical field. Many people (maybe you?) get so discouraged they just give in to the negative messages. Don't let that be you!

Like most people, have you ever known what to do (like diets, exercise, wise choices for any number of things), but find yourself avoiding, dragging, resisting, or just not understanding why you don't make progress?

The more you know about what stops you, the easier it will be to defeat it and gain a victory. I'm going to share some basic health information and the unseen things that undo whatever progress we think we're making. I'm also going to share some simple steps to turn that around. It's simple, but it may not always be easy.

However, it will be worth it if you decide you don't want to be diabetic anymore.

We'll cover the myths people believe. We're bombarded online and off with information about miracle cures. The food and drug industries block our progress in the name of profits. And then, of course, there are those pesky white lies (excuses) we tell ourselves.

I won't pull any punches or sugar coat it (sorry for the sugar reference already). There are terrible side effects of diabetes. There are ways to mitigate or reverse it if you do what is best. If you don't, you'll eventually live a lesser quality, shorter life.

If you want to get past your struggles, procrastination, or the things that stop you from making the progress you want, this is the book for you.

By understanding the issues underlying diabetes and prediabetes, you will be able to improve your overall health, plus discover a rewarding ripple effect throughout your life and that of your entire family.

If you're not diabetic but have a loved one with diabetes, this information will help you gain insight into their challenges and solutions. The information and understanding you'll gain will help you prevent your own possible diabetes diagnosis in the future. When you get involved with the healthy changes of your diabetic friend or family member, both of you benefit. Teamwork really makes everything easier.

In its simplest form, overcoming diabetes will require a decision on your part backed up with action. Often, it's a struggle you'd rather not have to go through. That's why you haven't overcome it yet. But overcoming disease is always worth it.

There are dozens of books on habit changes, willpower, self-management, and recipe books zeroing in on any number of food fads. Just like there are thousands of diabetes-related books. This one embraces both mind and body.

If you're like me, you don't read just one, but add knowledge bit by bit. I have a physical library full of such books and a growing number of digital books and audiobooks.

Each book adds a piece to our complex human puzzle and speaks to different people in different ways. Some become the "aha" and the words jump off the page, like the information about our brain did for me. You have something actionable. It's the "now I get it!" moment. I hope this book will do that for you.

> We're confronted with an incredible amount of hype and sabotage. This means we have internal and external influences that affect our progress in overcoming diabetes.

2

Our Lives Changed Forever

It was a Friday in 2009. Little did I know my life would change. My husband's already had.

What we thought was his routine medical checkup brought unexpected and unwanted results. The doctor suggested he also visit a heart specialist.

A series of four tests were scheduled, each a week apart, starting on Monday. While he was there on Monday, I got a call about the blood tests results: type 2 diabetes! I could hardly believe what I was hearing. I was scribbling down information, but my mind was swirling with questions and disbelief.

Meanwhile, the heart doctor was moving the second test to Tuesday. On Tuesday, the third test was moved to Wednesday. After that test, the doctor told him he needed an angioplasty. The procedure would insert a camera into his heart to see the condition of his arteries. If nothing more was required, he'd go home after the procedure. If it was necessary to insert the surgical balloons (stents) to open blocked arteries, he'd stay in the hospital overnight.

One week from his first appointment, he had four heart stents, a grim diagnosis, and a handful of prescriptions.

The only medical advice he got was to take the drugs, eat "better" and cut down on fats. He was advised that diabetes, plus the drugs and "inevitable" side effects, would ultimately kill him. Just keep taking the drugs to slow down the progression. We changed doctors. Twice.

I refused to believe the doctor's doom and gloom report that nothing else could be done to improve his health. I immediately started researching diabetes, including diets, health issues, medications, and side effects to find ways to regain a healthy lifestyle.

We'd been eating fast foods and didn't pay enough attention to healthy foods. We'd both gained weight. I changed the meals we ate. I decided if he couldn't eat something, I wouldn't either. It would be a team effort. With his permission, I became the food police. I was a good cop.

I read all the product labels and taught him to do the same. We knew we had to eliminate as much sugar as possible. As we worked our way through the grocery store one day, he looked at label after label and then bemoaned, "There's sugar in everything!" Yes, pretty much.

He took it seriously. He reduced his weight and ate more wisely. He was taken off the most dangerous drugs. He thanked me for saving his life with my research, saying if it were just up to him, he'd still be eating the wrong things and doing more unseen internal organ damage.

He urged me to write my first book, *Diabetes Diet Options: What to Eat, When to Eat and How to Regain Your Health.* I followed it up with the *Diabetes Journal* because tracking progress is very important.

He steadily lowered his A1C readings. His original A1C count was 9.5, which is in the danger range. After losing weight through smarter food choices, he also lowered his A1C to the normal range.

According to his doctor, he's no longer at risk of developing diabetic complications. He still needs to maintain good eating practices to make sure it stays in a healthy range.

Know Your Blood Sugar Numbers

Your fasting blood sugar is:

Normal: 70-99 mg/dL (milligrams per deciliter)

Prediabetes: 100-125 mg/dL

Diabetes: 126 mg/dL or higher

A1C Blood Sugar Chart				
	optimal	sub-optimal	normal	pre-diabetes
Hb-A1C	**4.0–4.6**	**4.7–5.1**	**5.2–5.6**	**5.7–6.4**
		diabetes	harmful	dangerous
Hb-A1C		**6.5–7.0**	**7.1–8.0**	**8.1–15**

3

Diabetes Basics

She's Now Prediabetic

My friend, Christine, told me she had her annual physical check-up, and her blood glucose count was 120. She's now prediabetic. I could hear the concern in her voice. Now what?

She's Now Diabetic

Betsy knew she was prediabetic, but she felt fine. Sure, she was a little overweight—okay, 40 pounds—but she had a family to take care of, work to do, and family meals to make. She ignored it since she didn't feel sick. She also ignored regular doctor visits, but eventually, she made an appointment.

She was stunned and angry at herself when her doctor said she was now a type 2 diabetic in the dangerous range. Her blood glucose level, triglycerides, and other blood test results were off the charts. He put her on insulin right away even though she was diagnosed as type 2.

He's Not Diabetic Anymore!

Recently Dan sought me out at an author event, excitedly sharing, "I'm not diabetic anymore!" A few months earlier we were discussing my book. He quizzed me about eating and food attitudes. He was prediabetic and didn't think he could reverse it. His doctor told him to expect it to progress to type 2, complete with all the health challenges that would happen over time. Once armed with new hope, he applied his new dietary information and got great results.

The More You Know

The more you know about diabetes, what it is and why it occurs, the better you will be able to make wise decisions about treatment, reversing it and living a longer, healthy lifestyle. The information doesn't have to be dry or boring.

Research shows that in 2017, 33 million Americans were diagnosed with type 2 diabetes. Of that number, an estimated 8 million people are undiagnosed. The number of adults living with diabetes continues to rise by 1.5 million people every year. That's 45 million diabetics by 2025 in the U.S. alone.

Latest figures from Public Health England indicate that 3.8 million people in England aged over 16 have diabetes. More than 1 million people are thought to have undiagnosed type 2 diabetes. This is around 9% of the adult population, with an estimated £14 billion being spent annually on treating the illness and its complications.

According to an American Diabetes Association study in 2012, people with diabetes spend 2.3 times the amount of money that people without diabetes spend each year on their health. That's $13,700 a year per person, about $7,900 of which is directly attributed to diabetes.

Most people are familiar with Type 1 and Type 2 diabetes and even gestational diabetes. But there are distinct differences plus other types as well.

Prediabetes

With a staggering 86 million Americans who are prediabetic, that's one in three adults! Most of them have no idea that they're in this group. Prediabetes simply means that blood glucose levels are higher than normal, but not yet high enough to be called diabetes.

These individuals are more likely to develop diabetes within ten years and are more susceptible to heart attack and stroke.

There are usually no symptoms, although being overweight is a clue. It's difficult to know for sure if you're in this group unless you're tested for diabetes and your numbers fall in the prediabetic range.

If so, you should be tested every year or two and make any needed lifestyle adjustments. If you're overweight and don't exercise regularly, you're probably at risk.

It might be better to call prediabetes by a more startling, but effective, term. To use cancer terminology, prediabetes is really Stage

1 Type 2 diabetes. If you look at it as Stage 1, it's a wakeup call. You can do something to reverse it before you get a diagnosis of Type 2.

Type 2 Diabetes

Type 2 diabetes is the most common type and results from insulin resistance, a condition in which cells fail to use insulin properly. Most people are diagnosed after the age of forty. A growing number of children are being diagnosed with type 2 every year. This may be the result of increased overweight among young people.

Those who are undiagnosed have all the risks. But they don't know they could be doing something to prevent irreversible damage that might even include sudden death!

Type 1 Diabetes

Type 1 diabetes results from the body's failure to produce insulin, and currently requires the person to inject insulin or wear an insulin pump. It is considered by some to be an autoimmune disease. It is not a lifestyle disease. Type 1 still responds to better health habits and exercise, often lowering the amount of insulin needed. However, this book is focused on type 2 and prediabetes.

Type 3 Diabetes

Type 3 diabetes, also called brain diabetes, is marked by memory deficits and a dramatic decline in cognitive function.

Researchers discovered in 2005 that the pancreas isn't the only organ that produces insulin. The brain also produces it. It's the key to your brain cells use of glucose, which is needed for their survival and normal brain function. It's now linked to the onset of dementia and Alzheimer's.

For some reason, this information hasn't gone much further than medical journals or an occasional health report. It shows up in blood sugar readings, and most conventional doctors continue to label and treat these symptoms as type 2. We see this demonstrated in statistics like "60% of type 2 diabetics have an increased chance of developing Alzheimer's."

Functional and integrative professionals are starting to pay more attention to type 3.

It's important for the patient to realize that he can improve his chances of avoiding dementia or Alzheimer's. While medications may vary, the same brain healthy foods and exercise apply to both type 2 and type 3.

Type 3c Diabetes

Type 3c diabetes adds to the confusion. Not brain related, it's caused by damage to the pancreas from inflammation, tumors, and surgery. It damages the pancreas and impairs its ability to produce insulin, digestive enzymes, and other hormones.

People with type 3c diabetes are twice as likely to have poor blood sugar control than those with type 2 diabetes. The onset of type 3c may occur several years after an injury to the pancreas.

Misdiagnosis has been common, which negatively impacts treatment. Nerve, eye, and kidney damage are possible consequences of this misdiagnosis.

Gestational Diabetes

This occurs when pregnant women without a previous diagnosis of diabetes develop a high blood glucose level. It may precede the development of type 2 diabetes, although it usually reverses after delivery.

From Food to Fuel – or Fat

Our food is converted to glucose and moves into the cells throughout the body to fuel all our energy needs. Cells require glucose for their cells to process correctly.

Insulin, created by the pancreas, is the key that opens cells to accept glucose and allow the proper absorption of nutrients and flushing out the toxins. The pancreas is a small organ hidden behind the stomach that produces hormones, including insulin, and enzymes to help with digestion.

When this capacity is limited or breaks down totally, it affects the amount of glucose (sugar) in the bloodstream.

Our bodies contain a little over a gallon of blood circulating from head to toe through our bodies. It is designed to contain a total of only one teaspoon of sugar.

If our blood sugar rises by even ¼ teaspoon, we go from normal to prediabetic! If it rises rapidly to one tablespoon (3 times the normal amount) it results in hyperglycemic coma and death.

To safeguard this, when we have a change in blood sugar, our body will do whatever is necessary to stabilize and protect us. The excess glucose is turned into fat.

Not as well-known is the fact that insulin regulates fat storage. It tells our cells to store energy, either as glycogen or fat and prevents fat cells from releasing fat for energy.

It tells the body to stop burning its fat stores and instead, absorb some of the fatty acids and glucose in the blood and turn them into more body fat.

The pancreas may slow down insulin production in this situation. Too much glucose left in the blood creates a toxic environment. Your blood sugar spikes and causes an insulin reaction.

The body continues to burn fat, but this causes the liver to make more and more ketones and ketoacids. The increasing levels make the blood highly acidic, which can become an emergency.

Most diabetes definitions indicate that the pancreas isn't producing enough insulin and that more insulin is needed so the cells can accept more glucose.

However, new evidence shows a different story. People are simply eating way too many carbohydrates, which is immediately converted to glucose. The cells have already accepted so much glucose that they're saturated and simply can't take in any more. The pancreas's insulin key stops working. More insulin isn't the answer.

The liver turns the extra glucose into fat. Unfortunately, it's attaching that fat to your vital body organs around your belly. This is known as visceral fat. You'll see health articles and fitness trainers calling this belly fat the most dangerous kind of fat.

The cells have already accepted so much glucose that they're saturated...The liver turns the extra glucose into fat. Unfortunately, it's attaching that fat to your vital body organs around your belly.

Diabetes Symptoms

Symptoms can be elusive, but here are some things to be aware of.

- Excessive thirst
- Blurry vision
- Frequent urination
- Being tired, lack of energy
- Wounds slow to heal
- Tingling hands and feet
- Excessive hunger
- Excess weight gain or weight loss (The kidneys work overtime eliminating excess as urine.)
- Itchy skin
- Yeast infections

- Numbness in fingers (With high blood sugar, the fingers and toes tend to lose circulation due to blood vessel constriction.)
- Sweet smelling urine, excess sugar in the blood
- Sweet smelling breath
- Irritability
- Frequent headaches (Usually headaches signal some form of dehydration and electrolyte problems, but it can indicate glucose problems as well.)
- Dry or cracked skin. (Dry skin could mean that the sugar in the blood is preventing water from reaching the skin's surface.)

Consequences of Taking No Action

You already read that millions are totally unaware they have diabetes. Because it can go unrecognized and untreated for years, by the time someone gets a diagnosis of prediabetes or type 2, they might already be on the slippery slope toward the side effects. Some are life-threatening, others are life-altering, and all are expensive.

A friend of ours was diagnosed with diabetes several years ago. He took his $700 monthly prescriptions but paid no attention to diet and lifestyle. He didn't see any point to doing anything about it because his doctor told him there was no cure. After a few years, he was declared legally blind, totally affecting his ability to do his job.

Since blindness is a side effect of diabetes, he might have been able to make lifestyle changes to prevent it or slow it down. For him, it was less about the physical progression and more about believing the doctor's doom and gloom message plus the mindset that kept him from acting.

Overweight is also an issue common to most diabetics and prediabetics.

You've probably thought about getting in shape, you've even read about different solutions, most of which either offer instant, no-effort-on-your-part options or lay out a complex system for totally changing your life.

Some sound too good to be true and probably are. Others require you to drastically change your eating habits and menu. *No thanks, you think.* That's when you get stuck and reach for that double cheeseburger and fries. Counter-productive.

Consequences and Side Effects

1. Diabetic coma
2. Overweight and associated health hazards
3. Compromised physical circulation
4. Headaches
5. Liver failure
6. Respiratory infection and sinusitis
7. Increased aches and pains
8. Lack of exercise (usually tied to overweight)
9. Blood sugar testing gets old fast, frequenty ignored
10. Ulcers
11. Sores don't heal properly
12. High blood pressure
13. Heart issues (doubles risk of cardiovascular disease)
14. Damage to blood vessels
15. Fluid retention that might lead to heart failure
16. Risk of pancreatic cancer*
17. Fatigue
18. Depression
19. Anxiety disorders
20. Infections
21. Compromised immune system
22. Side effects of medication
23. Hypoglycemia
24. Organ failure such as liver, heart, pancreas, kidney
25. Cancer
26. Increasing costs of meds and doctors
27. Blindness
28. Limb amputation
29. Erectile dysfunction
30. Dental issues
31. Possible loss of job (complications prevent doing the work needed)
32. Increased aging (yes, diabetes contributes to this!)
33. Inability of getting more (or any) life insurance
34. Medical insurance issues
35. Overtired, but often can't sleep
36. Confusion, mental fog
37. Dementia or Alzheimer's disease (60% of diabetics affected, 19% more women)
28. Premature death

* If your diabetes has been well-controlled, but you suddenly can't control your blood sugar, it may be an early sign of pancreatic cancer. Be sure to have it checked out immediately.

4

Lifestyle Choices

Disease does not occur unexpectedly,
it is the result of a constant violation
of Nature's laws.
—HIPPOCRATES

Diabetes is labeled a disease. Some people view diseases as something they catch, like the flu, or something they believe they can't do anything to prevent, like cancer or heart disease. Some think it's an inevitability because "it's a gene my family has." There is no diabetes gene.

More accurately, diabetes is a condition, or a group of symptoms, that have a name. But it's really a lifestyle condition.

It's a myth that a family history of diabetes means you will inevitably get it too. Instead, family history should be a warning to take better care of your health.

It's not genetics, but you might have adopted the eating and exercise patterns you learned early in life. You might be passing them on to your children as well.

It's still lifestyle choices.

You've heard that you should make changes toward a healthier lifestyle, and possibly you need to take off some weight.

You can start to align your body to absorb what it needs, understand what is happening on the inside, and prevent degenerative progression. But sometimes things don't work out as you hoped.

If you're like most people, you get totally discouraged and maybe even angry. Emotions are welling up. You've been hyped. You experience defiance or fear.

- *Why me? What have I done to deserve this?*
- *Am I going to have/be (pick any side effect)?*
- *Why isn't there an easy plan?*
- *What if I hate all that organic greens stuff?*

Your thoughts ramble from "Unfair!" to "It's too hard!" or "I just don't feel like it!" to "I don't like that food!"

You grow more resistant or settle into mind-numbing apathy. You don't know what to do, what really works.

Your doctor told you nothing will work, so you feel defeated before trying.

Maybe you're new to this, and you're uninformed about what is healthy and what isn't. And why. Who can help you? You're confused by so many contradictory voices.

- *"Why are so many people talking about organic everything?*
- *Is it really that important?*
- *Fast foods...what's so bad about that?"* Plenty, but we'll deal with that later.

You rationalize that you just don't have enough willpower. Your self-esteem plummets when you do try and don't have great results.

Maybe another rationalization (excuse) is that it's simply too expensive to eat healthy foods. How expensive are your increasing medicines? How expensive is it to be hospitalized, go blind, lose a limb? You get the point. There are less expensive food answers.

Maybe you believe you just don't have time to focus on making special meals. Or your family doesn't support you. "They keep all the wrong foods right there in the pantry and the fridge."

Then there's the boomerang effect. You try, but you can't keep it going. Bad habits keep coming back like a boomerang. You think you're just stuck with bad habits.

Then there's the problem of cognitive dissonance. This means you have inconsistent thoughts, beliefs or attitudes. You unconsciously have two opposite beliefs and they cancel each other out. Or it's two independent beliefs you've had for years. They didn't matter until you were diagnosed with diabetes.

- You believe you eat healthy foods
- You believe it's ok to eat out and have a couple of margaritas

In this case, your definition of healthy foods secretly means "except margaritas," or you're still feeling defiant.

The result is that you intend to do well, but you're self-sabotaging. "Oh no, not ME!" Sorry, yes, you.

The importance of this distinction: you can always choose to do something to improve your health and prevent the conditions from overtaking you. It does not have to be the doom and gloom often associated with it.

With this lifestyle disease, you should learn what you can do about it as well as what emotions are holding you back. When you learn the bigger picture, you can change a life sentence into a lifestyle worth living.

> When you learn the bigger picture, you can change a life sentence into a lifestyle worth living.

One lifestyle choice involves what and how much we eat. The fast-rising rate of type 2 diabetes among all ages can be linked to the rising rates of obesity. In 2015 diabetes was the seventh leading cause of death in the United States. That statistic is higher for children.

Diabetes focuses on the pancreas and the hormone it produces: insulin. Insulin is the key to open the cells to receive the glucose from our food. If the cells don't accept the glucose, it remains in the blood, resulting in high blood sugar.

Prescribed medications are intended to control our insulin production and blood glucose. Then we're told that some of those meds will adversely affect the heart, so we need heart meds.

Or by the time you get a diabetes diagnosis, you also have other medical issues that are common diabetes side effects over time. This was our story as my husband's diagnosis didn't happen until the heart damage was already evident.

Then the doctor tells you that after several years on the meds it could totally wear out your pancreas. That's pretty much as far as traditional medication goes (more on this later.) Doom and Gloom.

Health, emotional, and financial issues are often caused by the prescribed medicines themselves.

For some diabetics, some medications will continue to be necessary, especially when you already have other non-diabetic issues. For others (hopefully you!) taking responsibility for a healthier daily diet and exercise will produce dramatic results. Possibly even totally reversing your diabetes.

If you're like most diabetics, you want to overcome diabetes and prevent the other related challenges. Many people do that. Some people are still working on it but others let habits, myths, and excuses stop them.

I'm assuming you are in the "working on it" group.

First, the problems and solutions are not isolated to the pancreas. Your body is a unified, intricate system and your brain is the command center.

You have an ideal command program installed, and you have the Con. You get to decide what direction your ship goes, and if you are going to keep maintenance low and great adventures high.

Avoid The 4 Deadly Whites

1. Sugar
2. Rice
3. Flour
4. The White Lies you tell yourself about your health

5

Not Be Diabetic Anymore!

Intelligent people are always ready to learn.
Their ears are open for knowledge.

—PROVERBS 18:15, NLT

You have a diagnosis. You can simply shrug it off as inevitable, although if truth be told, you're probably scared, angry about it, disappointed at least. But don't stop there. You still have the chance to change your future.

You are not defined by career, a role you play in family life, or what your medical condition might be. You are a person who has a medical condition called diabetes. You can treat that.

No one else has a fingerprint exactly like yours. You're uniquely created to leave an imprint on the world that no one else can do. Your world might be global or as small as your immediate family. What you do with your uniqueness is up to you.

We each have been given free will, with the power to choose at any time in life to go this way or that, down a dark path or break out into the sunshine.

Your brain has been programmed unconsciously throughout your life by the circumstances and events of your life. This includes your thoughts and beliefs about your health and your future. You can step in and take charge.

You do that by changing your focus and doing some reprogramming. You 2.0.

Examine where you are now and how you got there. There's a book by Marshall Goldsmith, *What Got You Here Won't Get You There,* that clearly demonstrates that where we are is the result of the knowledge and experiences we've had so far.

But we must get new information, and willingly choose to upload that new information to take us in a better direction.

I've asked diabetics what they really want, and repeatedly I hear "not be diabetic anymore." Most likely, that's you too.

The good news is diabetes prevention and reversal is proven, possible, and powerful.

But perhaps you don't know what to do about it or how/why the side effects happen.

You want it all now, without much effort, and you want instant results! We all want that. Unfortunately, it doesn't happen that way.

You can overcome your diabetes, or at least dramatically improve your lifestyle. If you're just starting to make changes, it will be a struggle as you sort through the things you're doing to compromise your health. Many of them are things you've never thought about.

There's brain health, adequate sleep, what triggers our reactions, and the belief that we need more willpower. We also have an enemy in the name of hype and sabotage.

Start with some basics of healthy eating: maintain a healthy, well-balanced diet and reduce your intake of carbohydrates. Start or continue to exercise regularly. If you drink alcohol, reduce your intake, especially the sugary ones.

This is the starting point to keep your blood sugar levels as normal as possible. It's the beginning of reprogramming your health to prevent the side effects from that dreaded consequences list.

Your goal should be to have your doctor wean you completely off the medications.

They cause more negative side effects than they really cure. If you are doing all the healthy steps to regain your health, you should be able to stop some or all medications.

The reality may be that there are heart or other related side effects that require some medication, but if you get started soon enough, it may be possible to become completely drug-free. Be sure to check with your health care provider and do not simply stop taking prescribed medicines.

Become more active and make changes in what you eat and drink even if it seems challenging at first. You may find it easier to start with slight changes and get help from your family, friends, and health care team. It's not all-or-nothing!

That sounds good, but most people find it difficult to follow through without help or understanding what really stops them.

Everywhere you look it's "do this, do that!" Every day things come out in videos, magazines, books, and blog posts. So, how seriously do you want to be well? Only you can answer that.

If you're like me, those things that frustrate you may be the very things that you sometimes do. And when frustrated, we may do more of those things that frustrate us. Go figure!

We're not alone in this frustration, nor is it something new. Over 2,000 years ago one of the most well-known leaders, Paul, was sharing his own struggles in letters to his followers.

He wrote about this very thing. *"I have the desire to do what is good, but I cannot carry it out. For I do not do the good I want to do, but the (bad habits) I do not want to do—this I keep doing."* —Romans 7:18-19, NIV.

He didn't let that stop him from reaching his goal of continuous improvement. *"Forgetting what is behind…I press on toward the goal to win the prize."* Philippians 3:13, NIV. He offered encouragement, too. *"Let us not become weary in doing good, for at the proper time we will reap a harvest if we don't give up."* Galatians 6:9, NIV.

It takes time, but commitment and consistency will bring the results. The effort you put in will pay off richly in the end. It will require effort and a mindset decision about what's possible.

Visualization: Imagine Overcoming Diabetes

Sit back and imagine with me that you've conquered all the obstacles you faced that held you back from overcoming diabetes.

How would you feel as you get dressed each morning? Looking at yourself in the mirror brings a smile to your face. You notice your clothing fits better. Or maybe it's time for a shopping trip for new clothes.

You don't wonder or worry about the side effects of diabetes anymore. Every checkup shows an A1C in the normal range. You're not at risk of those complications anymore. You have more energy, and fewer aches and pains.

Your initial worries that eating healthy would be too expensive are totally gone. In fact, your budget has expanded because you have fewer medical expenses.

Family interactions are easier somehow. You're participating in activities that used to be stressful for you. The brain fog that plagued you is gone.

You're getting your work done with less fatigue as well. Oh, sure, there are still those other employees (or family members) that we all deal with, but even that's easier to cope with.

Imagine that you have improved your career options. So much easier without the debilitating side effects to worry about, isn't it?

Now think about what really thrills you. What would you love to do?

Where would you like to travel? As the commercial says when the team wins, we're going to Disneyland!

Dream as much as you wish. Take your time and really feel how winning this fight will be.

Visualize for a few minutes every day to stay focused on the results you want.

6

Note to Non-Diabetics Who Love Diabetics

A mind changed against its will
is of the same opinion still.
—BENJAMIN FRANKLIN

If you're the loved one of a diabetic and you aren't diabetic, it will be important for you to understand the struggle that might be going on about making healthy lifestyle changes.

You might even want the changes more than they do. You can't force someone to change. Certainly, don't try to intimidate or cajole them, which is pretty much guaranteed to fail. The diabetic must want the changes for his or her own reasons, not yours.

When it's not your personal health problem, it's easy to have answers to fix things. But you can't fix other people. Only they can do that. If they don't want to, you'll see conflict instead of agreement.

You can only encourage them, gently. No lecturing. Otherwise, resistance will set in. "Oh no, not me." Their self-talk will justify their current habits and cast you in the role of someone who's never satisfied, uncaring, or other negative thoughts to compound their justification process.

The fact that you genuinely care about the other person is completely lost on them.

And each person processes information in a different way. For example, my husband's communication style is very much the thinker and contemplator (opposite mine). He will think through any situation complete with, "If I say this, she'll respond with..."

A positive shift came for us when I noticed him staring nowhere and asked if he was having a mental conversation with me. "Yes."

"Am I responding?"

"Yes."

I kept a casual tone and said, "No fair. I'm not there to defend myself. Maybe I wouldn't respond as you think."

He speaks up now, and our relationship is even better since we communicate out loud.

I'm sure he still has mental conversations, but we have a foundation for not making assumptions.

He also taught me a lot about how to present the facts at the right time and in a kind way so that he can process them on his own and make wise decisions. I have to give him the time needed to process.

2

PART

7

What Stops Us?

So, what gets in the way of success? Turns out it's pretty much the same as what stops us in anything. While I was specifically looking for things that affect diabetes, I discovered it includes a lot of truths beyond diet or exercise.

There are the myths we believe, the limiting beliefs that hold us back, the excuses we make. We're assaulted with hype and sabotage from the medical and drug industries. Unfortunately, some sabotage comes from friends and family. Or self-sabotage.

Making a decision to change a lifestyle habit is the easy part. Follow-through, not so much. Millions of New Year's resolutions are made but abandoned in short order.

Procrastination and other bad habits overwhelm us. Even when we have great intentions.

Well-meaning doctors share death-sentence messages about diabetes. They are following their limited conventional training.

Online messages tell you about the latest discovery that solves your diabetes forever, but only with their special product. Just enter your credit card info.

It's information overload! What and who should you believe?

One book, article, video or report tells you to do one thing, and the next advises you to do something totally different. You're wading through good information mixed with hype and half-truths to get to the best and healthiest answers. New discoveries are made, and more information gets written. It's like being on a merry-go-round.

Life events may take you off course. Perhaps illness, depression, family struggles, finances. Or weddings, babies and birthday parties.

Temptation shows up at events. It can be so easy to say you'll just nibble a little, which turns into eating a lot.

Why? Our brains are hard-wired to resist change unless it has enough information to recognize a better way (like knowing why you really want to accomplish this.)

Some people easily embrace change. Most resist just about anything that sounds like change.

It's possible that you might have some resentment about 'having" to eat in a way you just don't want. Maybe you were forced to eat your vegetables before you could leave the table as a child (yuck!

Brussel sprouts!) So now you might subconsciously resist being told what to eat. It happens.

Or perhaps your belief has been that getting healthy is for everyone else, but not you. This is a common thought, but it's not true. If it works for one, it works for anyone who gives himself permission to succeed.

Give yourself permission to take down the protective walls that hold you captive. One brick at a time.

Do you need a mindset pivot to go from discouragement to hope in order to manifest your desired results? You'll find ideas and encouragement in the following chapters.

Don't go it alone. Find someone who understands your diabetes journey and can help you navigate the process. You need a cheerleader as well as an accountability partner. Sometimes it's the same person, sometimes a group, or a couple of individuals who each provide significant help for you.

8

Myths

Let's look at some myths that you might unconsciously believe. Knowing the facts will help you consciously move away from limiting beliefs and toward overcoming.

Myth: It's genetics

Fact: A family history of diabetes does not mean you will inevitably get it too. Instead, it should be a warning to take better care of your health. You might have adopted the eating and exercise patterns you learned early in life. You might be passing your habits on to your children as well. It's still lifestyle choices.

You can break this cycle with better choices for yourself and your family. Have you ever observed a family in a restaurant where all the adults and the children are all obviously overweight? This isn't genetic but learned. Setting a good example for your children to follow is important. Most children are consciously or subconsciously tuned into their surroundings and will eventually follow what they observe.

Myth: I'm too old to do anything about it

Fact: It's never too late to eat better, get physically active and take your health seriously. Don't let anyone else cast a life sentence over you. Someone saying "At her age, she's not going to change" leads to thinking you can't, so you don't even try. Know that you can change.

"You are never too old to set another goal or to dream a new dream." —C.S. Lewis

Myth: I've had this too long for anything to change

Fact: It is never too late to start. The rest of your life could be a long time. Now's a good time to choose your future.

Myth: That's just the way I am

Fact: Only if that's what you believe. Do you want to be better? It doesn't have to be that way. With good information and encouragement, you can be in control of a healthy lifestyle.

Myth: God wants me to have diabetes.

Fact: If someone told you this, he/she was mistaken. There is no place in the Bible that indicates it's God's will for you to be diabetic. Instead, it's his desire for us to be well. It isn't a punishment. More likely, it's the consequence of life choices over time.

Myth: If you're overweight or obese, you will eventually develop type 2 diabetes.

Fact: Being overweight IS a risk factor for developing diabetes. But other risk factors such as eating patterns, ethnicity, and age also play a role. Some people disregard the risk factors and think that weight is the only risk. Many overweight people never develop type 2 diabetes, and many type 2 diabetics are at a normal weight or only moderately overweight.

Myth: Eating too much sugar causes diabetes.

Fact: The answer is not so simple. Type 1 diabetes may be an autoimmune disease. Unknown factors can trigger the onset of type 1. Type 2 diabetes, however, is a lifestyle condition.

Being overweight is a risk for developing type 2 diabetes and eating large amounts of calories from *any* source contributes to weight gain.

Research has shown that sugary drinks ARE linked to diabetes. The American Diabetes Association recommends that people avoid intake of sugar-sweetened beverages to prevent diabetes. Sugar-sweetened beverages include:

Regular soda

Fruit punch

Fruit drinks

Energy drinks

Sports drinks

Sweet tea

Flavored waters

Other sugary drinks

They raise blood glucose and provide several hundred calories in just one serving! One 12-ounce can of regular soda has about 150 calories and 40 grams of carbohydrate. This is the same amount of carbohydrate in 10 teaspoons of sugar! One cup of fruit punch and other sugary fruit drinks have about 100 calories (or more) and 30 grams of carbohydrate.

Myth: There is no cure

Fact: Logic should tell you that if anyone has been cured, there must be a cure. A growing number of people have adjusted their life choices and found a cure for their medically diagnosed diabetes. The debate seems to be with the words, "cure" or "reversal," which some people find easier to understand. And a cure isn't a license to go back to bad habits.

Myth: Diabetes is not a choice

Fact: You can do much to prevent prediabetes and type 2 in the first place. If you overeat, consume large amounts of sugar, and don't exercise, you are at risk. But that's still your choice. Type 2 can be reversed through diet and exercise.

Myth: Diabetes is not a serious disease.

Fact: Diabetes causes more deaths a year than breast cancer and AIDS combined. Having diabetes nearly doubles your chance of having a heart attack. The good news is that proactive diabetes control can reduce your risks of complications.

Myth: People with diabetes must eat special foods.

Fact: A healthy meal plan for people with diabetes is generally the same as a healthy plan for anyone: low in saturated and trans-fat, salt and sugar, with meals based on lean protein, non-starchy vegetables, healthy fats, and fruit. "Diabetic" foods generally offer no special benefit. Most of them still raise blood glucose levels, are usually more expensive, and can also have a laxative effect if they contain sugar alcohols.

Myth: Diabetics eventually lose their feet.
Fact: Foot and leg problems are a concern for diabetics. If they are not careful to keep their A1C and other indicators in check, they may very well develop the side effects of diabetes. But it is not an inevitable process. You have considerable control of the outcome.

Myth: Diabetics can only eat small amounts of starchy foods.
Fact: Awareness is key. Starchy foods or carbohydrates are quickly turned to glucose. Many foods are genetically modified and are unhealthy for that reason. Some such foods can be part of a healthy meal plan, but portion size is key. Vegetables, fruits, beans, milk, and yogurt are also sources of carbohydrates. Choose low glycemic foods.

Focus on proteins and vegetables first. Cut back on sugars and carbs, especially when you first start a health program. Once you've established a healthier routine, you can start adding carbs back into your meal plan but be sure it's a properly sized portion.

Whole grain bread, cereals, pasta, rice and starchy vegetables like potatoes, yams, and peas may be included in your meals in small portions and less frequently.

Myth: Diabetics can't eat sweets or chocolate.

Fact: If eaten in small portions as part of a good health plan, sweets and desserts may be eaten by diabetics. The key is to have a very small portion and, preferably, save them for special occasions so you focus your meal on more healthful foods.

Do celebrate!

Myth: You can catch diabetes from someone else.

Fact: No! No type of diabetes is contagious. You can't catch it like a cold or flu. Lifestyle factors play a major part in prediabetes and type 2 diabetes.

Myth: Diabetics get more colds and other illnesses.

Fact: You aren't more likely to get a cold or another illness if you have diabetes. However, any illness can make diabetes more difficult to control, so you should maintain healthy eating, sleeping and exercise routines to build your immune system as well.

Myth: If you need insulin, you aren't taking care of your diabetes.

Fact: Type 2 diabetes is a progressive disease unless it is minimized, reversed or cured through healthy lifestyle choices. When first diagnosed, many people with type 2 diabetes can keep their blood glucose at a healthy level with oral medications. Without proactive action on the part of the diabetic, the side effects and deterioration of internal organs may result in the need for insulin to balance the blood glucose levels.

Myth: Fruit is healthy, so eat as much as you wish.

Fact: Fruit is healthy. It contains fiber and lots of vitamins and minerals. But many fruits contain high amounts of natural sugar or carbohydrates, which raises blood glucose. Talk to your dietitian about the amount, frequency and types of fruits you should eat. Check the glycemic index of fruits you like. Choose the whole fruit instead of the juice, which no longer has the fiber.

9

Excuses and Beliefs

Your brain is hard-wired to keep you safe. It hates change. Excuses are limiting beliefs that your brain uses to prevent changes that it views as threats. You can overcome this wiring with a consistent habit change plan.

Don't allow limiting beliefs to hold you back. Examine them for what they are: excuses. Once you recognize them, they may be simple to change. Some will take more effort and time.

Substitute limiting beliefs or excuses with positive, empowering beliefs. The brain can't stand a vacuum, so you must replace the limiting belief with another newer, positive belief. When you do this, the change becomes easier.

Here's a sampling of typical excuses.

It's not realistic

This is an excuse to not try. Roger Bannister broke the 4-minute mile by doing something others considered unrealistic. He set a goal to break that barrier although others warned him that his heart would fail him. After he did break that limiting belief, many others also ran a mile in 4 minutes or less.

I can do it by myself

This is true, but more difficult than working with a doctor, coach, or workout partner. Find a friend to join you on your journey. Having an accountability partner makes everything easier. If one of you slips the other is there to help him up and to encourage you on. Get a coach. Ask a friend if you can check in for encouragement.

It's too hard

Everything is difficult when you first get started. Was it hard to learn to drive a car? Or to learn how to play various sports, or sing, or even read? Start small, make a commitment to continue, and it will become easier. Not taking control of your health now will seem easier until you discover the damage to your body, your brain, and your ability to live an active life. That's hard, too.

> I hated every minute of training, but I said, Don't quit.
> Suffer now and live the rest of your life as a champion.
> —Muhammad Ali

Most of us won't need to train as Muhammad Ali did, but the principle is still "Don't quit." Your efforts will show that you are a champion, too.

It takes too long.

How long did it take to get where you are now? It's perspective. Take it one day at a time and set short benchmarks. Celebrate each victory. Also, think about how long you'll be stuck with side effects if you choose to do nothing. The rest of your life.

It's boring.

There are ways to make it more fun, not boring. Make it unique to you.

It's easier to do nothing

Yes, it is! But how's that working for you? While you do nothing on the outside, your body is deteriorating on the inside. Soon you will be forced to do things you really don't want to do. Review the consequences of doing nothing. The status quo is not the way to go.

I want an easy way to get fit.

Everyone does. But easy doesn't usually provide the desired results. Find a simple-to-follow food plan that preselects healthy foods and quantities. Track it daily. We worked with a meal plan that restricted all added sugar and allowed no fat for about 40 days. It was a jump start to weight loss and retraining the brain and the body about what foods were good and which were not healthy choices. It advised no exercise during this period of time. Some people consider that too difficult, but for those who do it, it's easy enough. It was a mindset choice at the beginning. Follow a healthy plan exactly to reset your appetite and health. The rewards are great.

I need to give up too much.

You can decide to give up poor food choices and instead choose healthy foods. What you will give up is excess weight, fatigue, money spent on fast food, and negative health issues. You'll also give up buying into excuses.

It's too expensive.

Some organic foods do cost more than non-organic. Choosing meats and other proteins that you fix at home may be more expensive than packaged processed food. But they're healthier.

Consider what you eat. Think about all the sandwiches, chips and desserts you consume every day and think about the cost of these things.

How much harm do you bring to your body on a regular basis with this type of diet? Think about a gradual shift to healthy eating: include more vegetables, salads, fish, white meat in your day-to-day meals.

You'll realize as you eat healthier, the cost of being unhealthy is far more expensive. How expensive is hospitalization? Prescriptions? Time lost from work? Not being able to participate in family activities? Shorter life span?

Long term, you'll save on medical expenses and restaurant tabs. Eating out is more expensive than eating wisely at home.

My family doesn't help

This may be true right now. It can be a very real part of the sabotage you face daily. They may be confused or angry, or don't know how to help.

It still isn't a good excuse for you to forfeit being proactive with your health. Perhaps you can share the chapter titled *Note to Non-Diabetics Who Love Diabetics.* Sit down for a family conversation and brainstorm ways to work together. A healthy lifestyle is good for everyone, not just the diabetic.

10

Hype

The more I've researched, the more I'm convinced it's not your fault. I used to think that statement was just permission or an excuse for not taking responsibility. Not anymore.

Marketers see an opportunity for profits. The food and drug industries are sabotaging us! The food industry adds and promotes sugar to keep you buying their products.

You've been set up to fail!

With all the health concerns and solutions blasting the airwaves, it's easy to get confused about what's good and what isn't. It's a catch 22.

Sometimes it seems easier not to make changes. That's when you might think, "Skip the workout and check the pantry for snacks. What's on TV tonight?"

Yes, you need to take responsibility for what you choose to believe and how you act to make the best of your health. But it doesn't stop there. There are so many outside influences confronting us every day. If you become aware of the marketing hype, you can overcome it!

The miracle cure hype is rampant. Marketers play on our old conventional wisdom that pretty much got us where we are now: overweight and unhealthy. As you'll also see in the chapter on sabotage, we have a lot to learn and overcome. It can be done!

It's a Miracle Cure! Or is it Hype?

Marketers have found an audience of individuals who desperately want a diabetes cure. The field is wide open for any marketer to promote diets, pills, books, miracle cures, and programs with excitement and even extreme hype that grabs your time and attention but won't tell you their answer until you take out your credit card.

They offer instant, no-effort-on-your-part options. Or a complex eating and workout system that, deep down, you're sure will hurt you.

They create elaborate, dramatic stories about finding a miracle cure. Of course, they claim they're the only ones who have it. It's only available for a limited time, and Big Pharma is afraid of them (no, they're not!) Supplies are limited (no, they're not) so order now.

You're bombarded with that magic diabetes cure or diet pill where weight just drops off your body while you sleep, or another that melts fat with no effort on your part.

You've been set up to fail!

What about exercise? Someone's promoting exercising for 7 minutes a couple of times a week as you go on with the rest of your life as usual. Another promotes a 45-second-per-day exercise as all you'll need to lose 35 lbs. Sounds easy enough. Just send $$ to find out what the workout routine is (after watching their 45-minute video).

Often the claims include taking their product and continuing to eat whatever you want. No, you can't. That's what got you here in the first place.

The challenge with miracle cures is that they're market driven (to make sales) and not to truly benefit the people who desperately want an easy, quick cure. They know people are willing to try whatever sounds good by pushing their emotional triggers. And they are skilled at pushing emotional triggers!

Thoughts you might be having about those miracle cures

- It looks easy
- They say my doctor is lying to me
- I'm so tired of not feeling good

- At least it's not broccoli
- Something has to work. Maybe it's this one.

Who are they? Most are marketers, not accredited medical professionals or nutritional experts. I've even recognized the voice of the actor (yes, actor) reading the messages as different doctors. Any actor can wear a lab coat, have a stethoscope around his neck, and read a script.

Am I saying they're all bad? Of course not. But you need the big picture and a plan first. Then you can see if what's promoted fits into your plan, or if it's just a reflex action to find an easy way to stop being diabetic.

I've watched dozens of videos and read numerous sales letters just to see if they're promoting something truly amazing or not.

Some are doctors with a viable product presented without hype. Most are not.

The writer of the sales ad, whether video or print, has included all the sales tricks to pull your emotional strings. They like the word "Warning!" indicating this video is so controversial that the conventional doctors or Big Pharma will shut them down as soon as they find the video.

No. They have bigger things to focus on.

And you "must order now" before the video disappears, or they run out of stock. They say they don't know if or when they can get more of the precious product. Of course, that contradicts urging you to select the auto-draft subscription for a shipment every 60 or 90 days.

Another thought: If they're such miracle cures and take only 21 days, why are they asking you to be on autoship every month? Or buy 3 or 6 bottles to save money per bottle. If you bought it, are you getting any benefits from it? Did the first bottle work?

Some so-called miracle cure products claim to have a newly discovered ingredient that will solve all your health issues.

Don't depend on that single ingredient without knowing if it needs other ingredients to perform as expected. If so, or if you fail to follow the directions completely, it will only be a miracle cure for the marketer's bank account. You'll get no real benefit.

I'm sure you've seen, read or even tried these miracle cures that proclaim you can eat a certain diet for just 21 days, or take an amazing, newly discovered pill without having to change what you eat. You're good to go, they say.

Some even suggest you'll astound your doctor and can throw away your medications.

Please don't fall into that trap!

No matter how wonderful the miracle cure is, the timing is simply unreasonable. Plus, if you don't know the various ingredients of the miracle pill or diet, it might have negative interactions with your brain and body. It can cause far more harm than good. You don't want to end up in the hospital!

Hype Cloaked in Half-Truth

I recently read an ad positioned like a news article that claimed scientists had discovered "something new" in the blood of all overweight people that "isn't there" for those who are not overweight.

Apparently, it prevents overweight people from *ever* losing weight "even when they do everything right." Snacking, stress eating, food addictions, binging, willpower, and other eating patterns have *nothing* to do with overweight, they say.

Several paragraphs later, we get the big reveal. The "something" is C-Reactive Protein (CRP) The truth is CRP is a *normal part of everyone's blood* and can be measured to see if we have excess amounts, indicating possible internal inflammation. If it measures *in excess,* it might indicate inflammation, which is common to overweight people. It does not mean you have no hope of losing weight.

While inflammation does play a part in weight loss, it's not as you might think. Sugar is inflammatory, and therefore causes inflammation and a chain of events that follow.

It may cause intestinal permeability and cause you to develop food allergies. It can initiate autoimmune diseases. The article, however, ignores all of these things and exclusively blames CRP. The real enemy is what you eat: sugar.

The truth is when we overeat or eat the wrong foods, it adversely affects three critical hormones: insulin, ghrelin, and leptin. Insulin is part of our blood glucose regulator, but it's also the fat storage hormone. If glucose is too high, the pancreas sends a signal to the liver to store the glucose as fat.

Ghrelin lets your brain know you're hungry. Leptin tells your brain when to stop eating. If insulin is too high, leptin is too low, so we keep eating. What and when we eat directly affects these three. Lack of sleep also affects leptin, which may be to why less sleep contributes to preventing weight loss.

The article doesn't mention these three hormones, or how they interact in our body systems. They even made up an official-sounding name, "weight loss resistance," as proof that it's not your fault. And they have the only solution.

Their solution is a supplement that you can only buy through them. That's when the news article becomes an ad pitching the product.

This is one of hundreds of articles, supplements, and dramatic stories meant to get the readers to buy their miracle cures. The marketing is aimed at the readers who want an excuse or a simple one-step solution.

Well-intentioned people who are trying to eat properly may be lured into this type of solution, just hoping it's a faster answer. If the reader is unfamiliar with the facts which might be omitted, it's easy to pull out a credit card and order. Autoship anyone?

There are products that do supplement your body's need for certain vitamins, minerals, enzymes. There is a growing group of doctors and researchers who formulate quality products and offer them without the over-the-top hype claims. But for the most part, the miracle cures aren't serving this purpose. They are profit driven.

I'm constantly getting emails and video pop-ups like "Cure Diabetes in 14 Days with This One Product." I've been added to way too many email lists. They are all written to create enough curiosity to open the email.

15 Email Subject Lines *(and my comments)*

1. 35 LB lost in 45-seconds with this "thyroid exercise"
2. Your shipping confirmation *(I didn't order anything)*
3. ¼ tsp of this bedtime spice kills flab
4. What's your address-sending you a cookbook *(wants me to order it)*
5. Surprising truth: #1 thing making us fat-not what you think
6. Canceling your order. Almost sold out *(I didn't have an order)*
7. How the Feds "stole" your health in 1954 *(actually some truth to that)*
8. Eat this oil before bed to burn 1-2 lbs. daily
9. Bad news for women *(Do I want to read bad news?)*
10. Study says this rivals antibiotics

11. 7 myth-busting arguments

12. Deadlier than obesity

13. Better than Law of Attraction. Fat burning trends

14. What _____ does to your body *(oranges, bananas, avocados, grapefruit, steak, fat, wine—you fill in the blank. It changes with each email)*

15. Bottoms up. Drink Tequila to lose weight *(promoting margaritas: apparently the type of sugar in their Tequila makes it okay for diabetics)*

The claims being made boggle the mind. They appeal to the results you want, but it could be dangerous or totally ineffective.

Here's part of an ad promoting an *only-from-us one capsule per day* cure:

- No more needles
- No more expensive and dangerous diabetes medications
- No more finger pricking or test strips
- No more trips to the doctor for discouraging test after discouraging test
- No more frustration and embarrassment
- **All in just 21 days.** *(emphasis mine)*

But wait! There's more! Sorry, couldn't resist.

11

Sabotage

We chat together; he gives me prescriptions;
I never follow them, so I get well.
—MOLIÈRE

Traditionally Trained Doctors

They are excellent at handling life-saving emergencies. Doctors are trained to find disease and manage it. But they haven't been trained to find the source of the problem. They work with bandaids on the symptoms.

Most truly care about health and healing, but they've had very little training during their many years of school. Your doctor finds problems and prescribes drugs. Only a small percentage of medical school courses even address wellness. This means he most likely doesn't understand how to heal, reverse or cure diabetes.

They focus on the drugs the pharmaceutical companies promote to control blood sugar. The sad fact is those drugs have toxic side effects that create bigger, more terrible health concerns.

Most diabetic drugs will eventually have a negative effect on your heart and other organs. Many eventually wear out your pancreas, heart, liver or kidneys. In fact, they do nothing to stop the progression of the disease. They mask the symptoms, which can lull the diabetic into thinking their health is better than it really is. At best, you're in maintenance mode.

One of the most common drugs is metformin. It prevents the liver from releasing glycogen into your bloodstream as glucose. This prevents your blood sugar from rising, but the diabetes is still progressing undetected at a cellular level. It puts extra stress on your liver.

Other meds put undue stress on the pancreas. When the drugs lose their effectiveness, doctors increase the dosage or prescribe additional medications. If the pills stop controlling the blood sugar, your doctor may put you on insulin.

Doctors continue to prescribe medication to manage symptoms, then add more to treat those side effects that come up, all the while telling the patient that this is all they can expect from life now. Seriously.

Unfortunately, some are truly Doom and Gloom dispensers, even though they don't mean to be.

Functional and Integrative Medicine

The doctor of the future will give no medicine but will involve the patient in the proper use of food, fresh air, and exercise.

—THOMAS EDISON

A growing number of professionals are proactive and seek prevention, care, and cure from diseases like diabetes. They are working against the sabotage.

Functional and Integrative medicine are gaining in popularity. Many believe it's the future of medicine. Doctors take a partnership approach with their patients, taking into account the lifestyle habits of a patient.

Their knowledge of health, what causes disease, what supplements or prescriptions will be needed, plus encouragement, couples with the patient's follow-through and feedback.

Integrative medicine treatments may include acupuncture, yoga or massage. They focus on nutritional and patient exercise to change habits related to obesity and diabetes. They look at poor lifestyle choices as the root cause of many diseases.

Functional medicine, like integrative medicine, focuses on supporting the whole person. However, functional medicine takes a systems-oriented medical approach to identify the root causes of a disease, particularly chronic diseases such as autoimmune and cardiovascular diseases as well as diabetes and obesity. Functional medicine is highly personalized.

Some doctors have forward-thinking practices and products. They may have YouTube videos and a following. Their products and training usually have sound science behind them.

Their patients are willing to invest in their own health and lifestyle, often without the advantage of insurance.

These doctors and health care providers recognize that the body is very good at healing itself, given the right foods and conditions. They seek to help patients find what works best for them. It's truly a partnership between the caregiver and the patient.

They can handle or refer out serious situations that do require critical care. They combine the best of alternative care and mainstream medicine.

Big Pharma is Vested in Profits

Most men die of their remedies, not of their illnesses.

—MOLIERE

Your wellbeing is not their problem. They research and create drugs that keep patients dependent on them.

According to John R. Lee, M.D., author of *Hormone Balance Made Simple,*

> "Most over-the-counter and almost all prescribed drug treatments merely mask symptoms or control health problems or in some way alter the way organs or systems such as the circulatory system work. Drugs almost never deal

> with the reasons why these problems exist, while they frequently create new health problems as side effects of their activities."

The sad fact is, most of the drugs have side effects that create bigger, more destructive health concerns. They know this. Most diabetic drugs will eventually have a negative effect on your heart. Or eventually wear out your pancreas, liver or kidneys. They have other medications for that, too.

Some clinical drug studies have been halted due to an increased death rate of participants. Some drugs with highly toxic side effects have been taken off the market. For those taking five or more medications per day, the risk of side effects is 50%.

There is a list of websites in the Reference section that monitor recalls, lawsuits and alerts.

Pharmaceutical lobby groups spent over $25 million in 2017, and that figure continues to rise. Each lobby group has an agenda to increase the profits of its own drugs.

Their focus? Provisions related to patent settlements, generic drug approvals, drug pricing, and importation. If they can slow down the release of generic versions of their drug, it keeps the profits in their coffers. The difference in cost to the patient between the brand and generic versions is mind-boggling, such as $500 vs $40.

Drug salesmen routinely visit doctor offices and hospitals with the latest industry news and products. Samples are given out and the medical field is urged to use their products. Most comply.

Concerns are now being raised over the influence the pharmaceutical companies have over FDA decisions and federal drug policy.

Beware of future diabetic vaccines. They still come from conventional thinking. They haven't been around long enough to check side effects, but what has surfaced lines up with conventional and not integrative/functional thinking.

Insulin: Did You Know?

- Taking more insulin just makes you fatter! It can also rapidly produce type 1 diabetes from type 2. Insulin is the fat hormone and works with the liver to turn your glucose into fat, usually belly fat.
- Acute deterioration of blood glucose control after administering insulin is a warning sign of this fattening problematic side effect.
- Additionally, increased insulin levels also
    - Make it virtually impossible for you to use your own stored body fat for energy
    - Suppress two important hormones: glucagon and growth hormone. Glucagon 35 promotes the burning of fat and sugar. Growth hormone is used for muscle development and building new muscle mass.
    - Increases hunger: as blood sugar increases following a carbohydrate meal, insulin rises with the eventual result of lower blood sugar. This results in hunger, often only a couple of hours (or less) after the meal.

Dr. Ron Rosedale, nutrition and metabolism expert stated,

> "Treating diabetics by overly raising insulin, either with drugs or insulin itself, is only further accelerating their aging, associated chronic diseases, and death, and should be considered malpractice."

Food Industry Sabotage

The food industry is also a player in this health crisis. They have corporate profits and shareholders to answer to. So, they do whatever is necessary to keep consumers buying their products. Because of marketing, the masses can be fooled into believing things are good for them but they are really not.

They constantly research what causes people to like and buy foods. They actually use the word *crave*. They want you to crave their products.

They spend millions of dollars on food lobbies to ensure that labeling and ingredients serve them, not the public.

Salt and the Food Industry

Salt is a key ingredient that the manufacturers wrestle with.

In *Salt Sugar Fat: How the Food Giants Hooked Us,* author Michael Moss stated a consumer group, the Center for Science in the Public Interest, carries massive clout in regulating advertising and how manufacturers label their products.

Frito Lay, for example, reviewed the Center's findings and created a specific study group to find ways to lower salt and still maintain flavor. They acknowledged that excessive salt consumption was a public health problem.

A research study done with monkeys concluded that salt and fat may contribute to higher saturated fat and higher cholesterol. But since no birth defects nor deaths were reported, they ignored the other health risk results in the study.

More than health, the financial bottom line was most important. They removed some salt to capture a more health conscious market, stating *"it would be wise to lower the salt content to **enhance sales.**"* (emphasis mine)

Fat and the Food Industry

Fat is a major component of processed food, a pillar ingredient even more powerful than sugar. Oils are all liquid fats, easily identifiable. Other fats are solid at room temperature and harder to distinguish. Cheddar cheese is one-third fat. Yet fats carry over twice the calories of proteins and carbohydrates: nine vs four per gram.

While not an obvious taste factor like sweet or salty, fat does contribute flavor. It also gives products long shelf life, can make cookies soft and tasty. Fat coats the tongue and hides the acidic taste of some foods.

Manufacturers continually experiment with how much fat to include for flavor, consistency and shelf life. Meats are classified by fat with ranges between 5% and 30% fat.

Fats don't blast our taste buds as sugar does, but it adds flavor when the sweetness is removed. When sugar goes down, fat is increased to maintain an acceptable flavor.

The balance of fats and sugar and salt are tricky business for food manufacturers because they do not want to hurt product sales. That is their primary concern in creating foods to market.

Fat-Free or Low Fat

In the 1980s, fats became evil. Fats didn't change. But the USDA and its experts wrote a booklet that sowed the seeds of the obesity epidemic. Their studies said fat is bad for you.

They didn't test all fats, nor did they check how the body needs and uses fat. They looked at one part of cause-and-effect and came up with unscientific conclusions, including the assumption that all fats caused cholesterol, heart disease, and overweight. Accordingly, they said we needed a diet virtually void of fats, saturated or mono.

There's a lot of flavor in fats. When they stripped out the fats, they had to add something to compensate for the flavor changes. Enter chemically created trans fats and sugar. They also created sugar substitutes, which have since been shown to have carcinogenic effects.

Trans fats and high fructose corn syrup became very popular in food manufacturing.

The rise in obesity coincides with this low-fat diet. All fats, whether healthy or unhealthy fats, were lumped together as bad.

Chemical and calorie rich substitutes soared. Margarine instead of butter. America bought into it and grew very fat.

Years later it's been proven how trans fats are poisons and, next to high fructose corn syrup, the deadliest ingredient in our food supply. There is no safe limit. There is no reason to eat them.

And still, conventional thinking takes a leap right past this obvious group of facts and conditions, calling it progress. The sugar and other food lobby groups were very active.

We now have a smarter view of what fats are good for us and which ones are harmful. The harm isn't only because it contributes to overweight, but because it eventually damages our internal organs.

It's been proven how trans fats are poisons and, next to high fructose corn syrup, the deadliest ingredient in our food supply. There is no safe limit. There is no reason to eat them.

Good Fats

- extra virgin olive oil *(without added canola oil—yes, some manufacturers add that to cut costs)*
- nuts and nut butter without added ingredients *(you can make your own in some grocery stores)*
- seeds like hemp, flax, chia
- fish *(see protein info)*
- avocado and avocado oil
- coconut and coconut oil

Fats to Avoid:

- all trans fats!
- hydrogenated or partially hydrogenated
- margarine and shortenings are trans fats
- butter, cheese, and full-fat dairy unless it's organically raised with no hormones or antibiotics
- factory farmed beef, pork, and poultry. Choose grass-fed, pasture raised
- vegetable oils with unhealthy omega 6. Do not eat soybean oil, vegetable oil, safflower oil, cottonseed oil or palm kernel oil

Food Trivia. How many did you know?

Fast food restaurants use yellow, red and orange because those colors stimulate hunger.

Corn dextrin is a common thickener in processed food and is also used as the glue on envelopes and stamps.

Average calories consumed at a buffet is 2,500. At a Chinese buffet, increase that average to 3,000 calories.

The FDA allows an average of 30 or more insect fragments and one or more rodent hairs per 100 grams (2 tablespoons) of peanut butter.

Americans consume the most ice cream in the world: 3.4 gallons (13 liters) per year per person. Most are consumed at night between 9 and 11 pm. Since some people don't eat ice cream, that means some eat a LOT more.

All carbohydrates that are not fiber will be quickly metabolized into sugar, which is like eating a large amount of sugar to keep your blood sugar lower. No, it doesn't make sense.

12

Sugar Is Your Enemy

Unfortunately, so are GMO's, processed foods
and non-fiber carbohydrates.
But let's focus on sugar.

Sugar is addictive, just like many drugs. Did you know that a brain scan of a person eating a lot of sugar looks virtually the same as a person on cocaine?

The commercialization and modification of sugar are destroying our health. It's virtually impossible to buy grocery store foods without sugar in some form. After all, there are profits and market share to consider.

The food industry is expert at knowing exactly how little sugar to add to keep its customers addicted to their products. Adding only the smallest addictive amount keeps consumers coming back and saves corporate profits. They even have a name for it: the bliss point.

They have been so successful that the average person consumes 71 pounds of sweeteners every year. That's 22 teaspoons of sugar per person per day.

> A brain scan of a person eating a lot of sugar looks virtually the same as a person on cocaine.

Adding carbs, such as flour-related products, gives a comforting texture to go along with the dopamine rush from eating.

The extent that they've gone to in order to keep consumers addicted to sugar is staggering. If you read food labels, you'll see that it's in nearly everything. In fact, it's in baby food. Start them early! Is it any wonder the kids don't want veggies and prefer all that sweet stuff? Childhood obesity is skyrocketing.

They create or modify products, calling them new and improved. The health food consciousness triggers the food industry to label products as healthy, like energy and granola bars. But a review of the ingredients shows they are loaded with sugar, although it may be in any of the chemical versions.

An examination of the ingredients of cereal reads more like candy. There's a reason the kids are hooked on Fruit Loops.

Sugar has many names: cane sugar, evaporated cane juice, brown sugar, dextrose, agave, maple syrup, honey, and of course, high fructose corn syrup (HFCS), which is now the single biggest source of calories in our diet. Plus, the chemical versions.

Most are chemically created and are meant to confuse the label reader. You might think there's no sugar in a product only to discover four or five different, unpronounceable ingredients that turn out to be sugar. If you add them up, it may turn out to be the #1 ingredient in the product.

Sugar-sweetened drinks like soda now make up 15 percent of the calories consumed by the average American.

It's in bread, ketchup, and salad dressings. In fact, the average serving of commercial spaghetti sauce has more sugar than a serving of chocolate sandwich cookies.

> "Sugar consumption is now an epidemic. The long-term effects will be staggering.
>
> —Mark Hyman, M.D., author of
> *The Blood Sugar Solution 10-Day Detox Diet*

A Short History of Sugar:
interesting facts you probably didn't know

Sugar use dates back thousands of years and was a tropical grass in southeast Asia. By 500 A.D. the people of India learned how to refine sugar cane into a powder which was used as a medicine to cure headaches, stomach aches, and impotence. The process was a closely guarded secret until it spread to Persia (modern day Iran). It was used by the rulers to provide sweets for their guests.

Around 600 A.D. Arab armies acquired the refining secret and spread the knowledge across the Arab world, according to *Sugar and the Evil Empire* by Geoff and Vicky Wells.

The Arabs perfected the sugar refining process, but the work was hard and hot, which they considered only suitable for slaves, primarily eastern European soldiers.

British and French crusaders, fighting in the Holy Land, were the first Westerners to discover sugar. Since their soil wasn't suitable for growing sugar, it was so rare that it was called a spice.

The spread of the Ottoman empire in the 1400s ended the sugar trade with the Arabs. The Portuguese began looking for a wet, tropical climate where they could grow sugar cane.

On his second voyage to the Americas in 1493, Christopher Columbus planted sugar cane in Haiti and the Dominican Republic. He'd been trained in the sugar trade. The Portuguese brought slaves to the islands to cultivate it. Sugar spread through Central and South America and was also exported to Europe to meet the growing demand.

Meanwhile, enterprising Europeans figured out how to extract sugar from beets, which they could grow easily in temperate Europe and North America.

Fast forward to the 1960s and 1970s when Monsanto entered the picture with chemicals to genetically modify the plants. Then came High Fructose Corn Syrup and other added sugars, most chemically created. High-fructose corn syrup consists of soaking corn kernels to extract corn starch and using enzymes to turn the glucose in the starch into fructose.

To make things worse, HFCS is made from GMO corn. This same corn fed to cattle makes them sick, so the cattle are injected with antibiotics, which end up in our burgers, steaks and other beef products.

Because of the growing backlash to High Fructose Corn Syrup, manufacturers changed HFCS to "fructose" or "fructose syrup" on labels. The original HFCS contains about 42-55% pure fructose, but the new fructose has been refined to contain 90% pure fructose. Buyer beware!

Countries that consume a diet high in HFCS or fructose have 20% more cases of type 2 diabetes than countries that do not.

64 Names for Sugar

agave nectar
barbados sugar
barley malt
Beet Sugar
blackstrap molasses
brown sugar
buttered syrup
cane juice crystals
cane sugar
caramel
carob syrup
caster sugar
confectioner's sugar
corn dextrin
corn syrup
corn syrup solids
crystalline fructose
date sugar
demerara sugar
dextran
dextrose
diastatic malt
diatase
ethyl maltol
evaporated cane juice
florida crystals
fructose
fruit juice
fruit juice concentrate
galactose
glucose
glucose solids
golden sugar
golden syrup
Granulated Sugar
Grape Juice concentrate
grape sugar
high-fructose corn syrup
honey
icing sugar
invert sugar
lactose
malt syrup
maltodextrin
maltose
Mannitol
maple syrup
molasses
muscovado
organic raw sugar
panocha
powdered suagr
raw sugar
refiner's syrup
rice syrup
Sorbitol
sorghum syrup
sucrose
sugar
Table Sugar
treacle
turbinado sugar
yellow sugar

3

PART

13

Results You Want

What health results do you really want? Do you want them now? Why do you want that? It must be why YOU want it for yourself, and not to please someone else.

If you want to be healthy so you can vacation with your family, you need to be doing it because YOU want that. If you really don't care about the vacation that involves so much walking, but you're making it your goal to appease their wishes, it won't be strong enough to keep you eating well when tempted or stressed.

Is your why big enough to help you power through those valleys that will inevitably come from time to time? Or to pull you back on track when you slip up? It happens to all of us. It's okay. But it's not okay to stay off track if you really want a healthy lifestyle.

Only you can decide if you want to make the changes needed to regain health or stay the same and live with the consequences. It can be hard to wrap your head around what changes need to be made. Decide you want good health more than you'll resist the process.

Are your thoughts on purpose or on autopilot? If you haven't had a plan for being healthy, then your non-plan has directed your actions. You've been on autopilot.

Today you can be the boss of your thoughts and choose to make them positive. If you're naturally inclined to see the glass half empty, that's workable, too. Whenever you realize you're thinking half empty, tell yourself *"cancel, cancel"* and substitute a more positive thought. Any tiny shift is good.

If you're living with someone who's personality is naturally negative, and you're the positive one, it might be a bit more challenging. Share your new health goals. Ask for their understanding and cooperation. Make it a team project. Most couples are personality opposites. Work to turn the differences into complementing one another, not disagreements and conflict.

What Habits Need to Change?

Which habit should you work on first? This will become your immediate goal.

The reality is you can't change everything at once. You'll get overwhelmed, discouraged and tempted to give up. Your brain will put up a fight.

Some people easily embrace change, but others resist anything that sounds like change. They are so comfortable in their habits that making any change to what and how they eat feels uncomfortable and causes resistance.

Some people can go cold turkey on eating habits. If you can, hooray! You'll see results sooner.

Most people need to pick one or two specific habits to change and add more as they start gaining success.

Once you commit to making changes, you can overcome your resistance. Accept resistance as a natural part of your thinking, but you can change those brain grooves.

21 days is neither scientific nor realistic.

You might have been told it only takes 21 days to change a habit. If you've ever tried for three weeks to change anything, only to have all your hard work vanish after that, it's easy to give up in discouragement.

It's just so easy to rationalize that you've done well for 3 weeks, and now it's time to treat yourself and celebrate with pie. Unfortunately, that thinking is not helpful! It's like an alcoholic going to the bar to celebrate a year of sobriety.

You'll probably return to your old ways, especially as it relates to losing weight. In fact, you might whistle right past the old weight and gain even more. That's just so discouraging!

If not 21 days, then how long will it take? Studies show that new habits are established in no less than 66 days and often it takes

90-120 days. So instead of three weeks and home free, you should plan on being consistent with the new habit you are trying to establish for a minimum of 66 days (two months). Three to four months is even better. By this time, your new, consistent actions become your new autopilot.

Let's say you know you should be careful about how much sugar you eat, but for 66 days you're going to eliminate all added sugar.

You'll need to break that into specific actions, such as learning to read labels and putting some foods back on the grocery shelves. Clean out the pantry and refrigerator to cut down on temptation.

Write out your goal, specifically stating the action you will take to bring the most benefit first. People with written goals have more success than those who just think about them.

Keep this in front of you on your desk, refrigerator or wherever it will remind you when you need it most. Focus on it daily. Visualize the success you were dreaming about in chapter 5.

Here are a couple of examples stated as actions you are taking and include your why:

- I'm cutting out sugar and adding veggies and protein to get healthy and feel better about myself.
- I read labels to avoid foods that contain added sugar.

Notice that you are focusing on something good instead of only eliminating something bad, which would create a vacuum. Your brain will try to fill it with anything. It hates a vacuum.

Tell yourself instead of donuts, you'll have eggs or an orange for breakfast. Instead of dessert, help clear the table. This is an action that diverts the mind. The alternative doesn't have to be another food option. Any positive action that substitutes for the one you are removing is helpful.

Focus on the new addition, not the one that's being eliminated. This is working smart, not hard. And you've elevated your thinking and increased your brain power.

You might be surprised by how your thoughts and your health are connected. Think healthy to become healthy.

You're training your brain, much like a bodybuilder trains his muscles, and increasing your intelligence, focus, and memory. Your mind is limitless. In fact, within three months you'll have a younger, healthier brain. The fact that it assists you in overcoming diabetes is true brain power.

Questions to Jumpstart Your Mindset for Health

- In the past, did you have bigger life plans?
- Have you settled for less because of your health? It doesn't have to stay that way!
- Do you really want to make changes? Why?
- Are you willing to act on those changes?
- Are you confused about what that really means?
- Assume you're now healthy and financially stable. How long would you like to live? Is it longer than you might have settled for in the past?
- Take some time to review the risks of consequences if you don't make healthy changes.

It's not comfortable in the beginning, I know. But it helps to get real with the possibilities and how they could affect you and your loved ones. It's never about only yourself but impacts family, friends, and career as well.

Dream. Dare to dream bigger.

Don't let others think for you. You decide. From there you can build toward your goal. There's no time limit other than how fast you want to go.

It does get easier.

Halfway-There Blues

As you progress toward your goal, it's not unusual to become discouraged at how long it's taking. We all want to go instantly from start to goal in a straight line, up and to the right. But there are so many other factors that turn it into hills and valleys. We can still arrive and win if we stick with it!

You could be halfway there, but you still have another 50% to go. This is the time to do a mental check of progress since you started.

Instead of struggling to see the finish line, turn around and look at how far you've come.

- You have a diagnosis you want to reverse
- You bought this book
- You gathered information about diabetes
- You decided on health goals, goal weight and learned what your healthy blood work numbers should be

- You discussed your needs and goals with doctor, family or friends for support
- You cleaned out the pantry and refrigerator
- You adjusted your food intake to the list of Foods You Should Focus On
- You shop with a list
- You chose some form of exercise you can stick with
- You bought a diabetes journal to keep track of your progress
- You visualize about the success you committed to achieve
- You tell a friend, accountability partner or coach if you need encouragement

You've come a long way, and it's worth continuing!

Next, we'll look at brain power, sleep, triggers and willpower.

How do they play into what stops you? What can you do to turn them into superpowers to accomplish your goals?

14

Brain Power

"As your weight goes up, your ability to think and reason goes down, which means that over time, if you don't get your weight under control, it will become harder for you to use your own good judgment."

—DR. DANIEL AMEN

You might have tried many things to proactively overcome your diabetes. And perhaps after a while, you've just given up and shrugged off your hope that things will get better.

But your thoughts can change everything.

Your brain is the control center for your entire physical system. It has 100 billion cells, more connections in your brain than there are stars in the universe, according to Dr. Amen, who has written numerous brain-related books.

Think of the brain as a computer with both hardware and software. Once you optimize the physical functioning of the brain (hardware), you optimize your mind (software).

It's only 2% of your body weight but uses 20% of the calories you consume and 20-25% of your blood.

Your brain is always thinking and talking to itself, which goes into your subconscious. This part of your brain handles self-talk. It can't distinguish the difference between fact and fiction, or negative and positive. It takes everything in as fact and reacts accordingly. You can use this fact to turn unhealthy thoughts and habits into healthy ones.

When people speak negatively about themselves, they unconsciously act in ways to prove those statements as fact, even though they may be far from the truth. If you tell yourself that you are fat, always tired, or can't exercise, then your brain will find ways to make sure you stay fat, tired, and prevent you from exercising.

If you mess up on something and say, *"Why am I so stupid?"* your brain will go to work to show you why you're stupid.

However, if you say, *"How can I prevent that from happening again?"* your brain will go to work to give you solutions to the problem. There will be no judgment about whether you are stupid or not.

If you tell yourself that you are fat, always tired, or can't exercise, then your brain will find ways to make sure you stay fat, tired, and prevent you from exercising.

The things we repeatedly say and do form habits, and 70% of our habits will determine how long we will live. So good habits result in a longer life than bad habits.

The brain is hard-wired to resist change. It's comfortable in the status quo, and therefore, you become comfortable in your good or bad habits. That's part of why it seems so hard to make changes. A change is seen as a threat and triggers the fight or flight response.

It sees this as avoiding loss rather than gaining something, and it keeps us focused on maintaining what we have rather than building something better or new. If you stay in status-quo, your life will continue to stay only the same, never to get any better.

Once you understand how habit creation and changes work, you can train your brain. But the thinking you've done so far got you where you are now. It won't get you to the next level. Learning this and consciously choosing your new thoughts and actions will bring the results you need.

"Do not conform to the pattern of this world, but be transformed by the renewing of your mind."

—Romans12:2, NIV

Your mindset is critical to success or failure. How you think about your new actions to reach a positive goal will make a difference in how easy or difficult the process will be.

If your brain has enough information to recognize a better way (like knowing why you want to accomplish this) it can overcome your resistance.

If you think something is being taken away from you, you'll resist. Instead of feeling deprived of desserts, salty snacks or sugary things, think instead that you're being given the gift of extended life by eating well.

Our habits are created through repeated input. This repeated action creates the equivalent of grooves in our brain, like grooves in records (old enough to remember them?) If the needle skips out of the track, it makes a jarring sound but settles into another groove.

Let's say you're in the habit of stopping by Dunkin' Donuts for coffee and a pastry or two on the way to work. You drive there without thinking, almost on autopilot. You're in the groove.

Now you have a desire to change to a healthier morning routine. The next day you deliberately skip your Dunkin' stop. Your brain has new information to process. Did you make a mistake? Is there a threat? Your fight or flight response kicks in. You did this on purpose to build a positive result, but your brain doesn't know that yet.

Off and on during the day, you might have thoughts of missing that donut. Push the thoughts away. Think of something more positive.

The following day you'll be faced with an urge to return to the old pattern. You'll need to consciously skip the donut stop.

Your brain is still resisting. It takes time to develop good habits. You need to break down your brain's resistance by repeatedly providing new stimuli. It will eventually replace the old groove, and your brain's routine will change to the new groove.

How long you've practiced the old habit will determine how quickly you adopt a new one.

Some habits will take longer. Your willpower plays a part, too (we'll discuss this in another chapter.)

Your brain is a supercomputer, but your heart works in conjunction with your brain. Many people believe that the communication is from the brain to heart, but doctors are more aware now that the heart sends more messages to the brain than the other way around. In fact, studies show that 90% of the messages move from the heart to the brain. That's partly why emotions are so important.

While our thoughts still control our feelings, any stress that we have in our mind affects our heart. That can determine how easily we can get healthy. Choosing to think positive, happy, grateful thoughts will push out the negative thoughts. This will increase the strength of the brain and reduce the body's stress levels.

Studies also show that we send and pick up signals from those around us. If you've ever heard of someone saying they had "bad vibes" from someone else, it's probably true. The positive side of that is the person who chooses to have positive thoughts will affect the attitude of others around him in a positive way. Mothers unconsciously sync their brain and heart rates to their children, especially when they are very young.

A stressed brain triggers tightened muscles that can shrink the grey matter of your brain. This leads to depression, auto-immune disease, insulin resistance, obesity, and insomnia. It slows down or stops healing.

Taking a few minutes at the end of the day to reflect on anything that went well, such as three things you're grateful for, will yield better sleep, and a better tomorrow. Thinking positive thoughts in the morning will start your entire day on the right foot. And it's contagious.

If you naturally fall into negative thought patterns or work in a stressful job, you might need to be more deliberate in pushing negative thoughts out and replacing them with thoughts of gratitude. You can even develop a routine to keep good thoughts in the forefront. Positive thoughts can become the norm that you can rely on.

How Choosing Positive Thoughts Overcame a Negative Diagnosis

Journalist Norman Cousins was diagnosed in 1964 with a degenerative disease causing the breakdown of collagen which left him in constant pain and unable to sleep. Doctors gave him six months to live. He refused to focus on the disease or side effects. Instead, he chose a positive approach. He checked out of the hospital and into a hotel room. He watched funny movies every day and took vitamin C and supplements. He said 10 minutes of deep laughter would give him 2 hours of restful sleep. He laughed his way back to health.

Brain Superfoods

We can help keep our brains active and young with foods that promote brain health. Here are some top picks. See also the chart Focus on These Foods.

Blueberries have been shown to shield the brain from stress, dementia, and Alzheimer's disease. Research has also shown that diets rich in blueberries significantly improved both the learning capacity and motor skills.

Avocados contain good, healthy fats, potassium, vitamins K, C and E, folate, iron, fiber, magnesium, potassium, B vitamins. These can improve your memory and concentration. They contribute to healthy blood flow and decreased blood pressure, lessening the chances of getting Alzheimer's disease or a stroke.

Broccoli has high levels of vitamin K which helps prevent Alzheimer's disease. It can improve memory and cognitive function as well as mood.

Leafy green vegetables slow cognitive decline with aging. Great source of vitamins A, C, E, K, and B vitamins, fiber, iron, magnesium, potassium, and calcium. Eat at least one serving per day.

Deep-water fish contain omega-3 essential fatty acids, which are highly concentrated in the brain and needed for healthy brain function. Wild caught only.

Nuts and seeds are good sources of vitamin E, an important vitamin needed by your brain to prevent declining cognitive functions. Cashews, peanuts, walnuts, sunflower, sesame seeds, and almonds are all great choices. Walnuts even look like mini-brains.

Complex carbohydrates supply the brain with a steady stream of glucose that enhances brain function. It's important to avoid simple carbohydrates often found in junk food because the glucose gives the brain a short-lived sugar high, often followed by a crash that makes you feel hungry and tired.

Green tea also has potent antioxidants that protect your brain from free radical damage and improve brain function.

Dark chocolate, eaten in small quantities, has powerful antioxidants, improve focus and concentration, and encourages the production of endorphins, which helps improve mood. It may help mental alertness, focus, and concentration. Other chocolates do not provide these healthy brain benefits.

15

Sleep

Eat well, drink in moderation, and sleep sound,
in these three, good health abound.
—LATIN PROVERB

Sleep habits and patterns affect overall health. How much you sleep affects your brain and how you process foods. Who knew?

Our most basic daily rhythm, the sleep-wake cycle, is related to the cycle of the sun. We should feel sleepy in the evening and wakeful in the morning. This is part of our circadian rhythms, ("circum" means "around" and "dies," means "day"). It's governed by our internal biological clock deep in the brain and the sun.

Melatonin is partly responsible for your body clock cycle. When there is less light, melatonin secretion signals the brain to shift into sleep mode and stops when the sun rises.

When we alter the sleep patterns of our biological clock we are more prone to health problems. The time shift for daylight savings times, jet lag and shift work all disrupt body rhythms. Hunger and metabolism, regulated with the biological clock, will be affected.

Two or more glasses of alcohol a day cause circadian disturbances that affect sleep, mood, body temperature, blood pressure, and hormone secretion. It also affects brain health through dehydration.

The brain needs six to eight hours of sleep per night to restore physical, mental and emotional reserves. During sleep, your brain is very busy at work, cleaning your brain, body organs, and body systems. It restores chemical balance, organ function, mood control, and willpower.

Toxins that have accumulated during waking hours are flushed by the brain back into the circulatory system and eventually to the liver where they're eliminated.

During the cleaning and repair process, 90% of your cells are replaced every 3 months, so this means you can have the equivalent of a new body every 90 days!

If you get an inadequate amount of sleep, this negatively impacts the brain's work schedule. Your biological clock is thrown off which then affects metabolism. Lack of adequate sleep also slows down or prevents weight loss.

Hunger, mental alertness, mood, stress, heart function, and immunity also operate on a daily rhythm.

Sleep weary people never seem to have much energy. There are numerous products such as energy drinks and supplements, gadgets, or motivational videos aimed to bring you more energy. The best way is just to get enough sleep in the first place.

> Sleep also affects your willpower. Since we wake with a certain amount of willpower, if we start the day overtired, we have less to start with.

How Our Body Responds to Sleep Schedules

Busy people often feel like there aren't enough hours in the day. So, they sacrifice sleep.

Whether staying up late to get more work done or to relax in the evening, less sleep compromises the body's ability to function properly.

Your reaction time and ability to process tasks efficiently will be impacted. You can catch up from a day or two, but if you've been short on sleep for more than a few days, it contributes to accidents and poor decision making.

If you're overtired and your willpower has ebbed away, it's harder to resist snacking, whether it's during the day or evening. Usually carbs. With sugar. Then regret sets in.

Science continues to discover important connections between a disrupted body clock and chronic health issues, from diabetes to heart disease to cognitive decline.

When you get more sleep, you'll see and feel positive results. After just one week, health benefits can include weight loss, joy, happiness, energy, and improved outlook on life.

If you're a shift worker, try to be as consistent with your sleep hours as possible. Blackout curtains for a day sleeper help. Getting adequate sleep is the most important part.

Sleep research confirms that people who rise early get more done. This isn't because they have more hours in the day since they also go to sleep earlier in the evening.

Many use the time for thinking, reading, and planning. Writers often use that time to write before going to their office job or getting the kids off to school. It's a quiet, undisturbed time.

Many night owls attempt to rise with the chickens. Some have more success than others. The ones who do claim great benefit from it.

If you want to try early rising, set your alarm 30 minutes earlier to start. When that time seems comfortable, move the alarm back another 30 minutes. Keep doing that in 30-minute increments until you're at your optimal rising time. If needed, do it in 15-minute increments.

When the alarm goes off, get out of bed. Do not hit the snooze button. You are breaking old habits and patterns. Create a new morning routine and do the same thing every day.

If you must work long hours on a project, do your best to still get six to eight hours of sleep each night. If you don't, brain fog alone will make the project drag on longer than expected, and more errors may show up.

Listen to your body: when it naturally gets tired, or how alert you are when you wake up. If you work well later in the evening, be sure that you still get enough sleep.

16

Triggers and Willpower

Making changes can be hard. We've been the way we are for so long, and it's comfortable. It may not be what we really want, but it's a habit. It's hard to initiate change, harder to stay the course, harder still to make it stick unless we are determined to make a change.

Inertia keeps us "as is" in our comfort zone. Until we have some reason big enough to make some changes. Diabetes and the potential consequences should do it. Sometimes yes, sometimes no. That's why we're here.

Triggers

Triggers are the reactions and emotions we have to thoughts, actions, and events in our past. Hearing a favorite song will trigger a memory of where you were when you first heard that song or the person you danced with when it played. Someone yelling at another may trigger a memory of being yelled at as a child.

We unwittingly shove these emotions into our subconscious, but the emotion surfaces when triggered. We might not even remember why. It's one of those programmed grooves.

To make a change, you need new information. You need to take new actions or think new thoughts to overcome a bad habit for a good one.

One benefit of visualizing yourself diabetes-free is that it speeds up the process of getting there. It's part of reprogramming your brain and collapsing the old triggers.

Make a movie in your mind where you have overcome your diabetes, or your shyness, or your ability to (insert your dream). You are the star. Others are proud of you. Take five minutes in the morning visualizing this.

One benefit of visualizing yourself diabetes-free is that it speeds up the process of getting there. It's part of reprogramming your brain and collapsing the old triggers.

This is what athletes do when they visualize each move on the playing field. They only see the correct choices, the correct move. Then when they're performing live, muscle memory and a winning program drive them on.

Your movie will do this for overcoming diabetes and anything else you wish to change.

If you're motivated but you don't know what to do, you usually do nothing. If you don't have your victory movie, buying into myths and excuses keeps you in your comfort zone. Learn what you need, what could stop you. then override the triggers that hold you back.

Excuses are explanations or rationalizations for why you failed at something after the fact. It's self-talk to assuage guilt and help you feel better. They are well-planned (but often unconscious) lies.

Our beliefs trigger failure before it even happens. They trigger denial, resistance, and self-delusion. Inner beliefs trigger the self-sabotage that stops us before we even get started. Then we use it to justify our inaction.

If you decide on a new course of action, but then don't do it, you trigger confusion. A confused mind says no.

Different actions can set off triggers that bring up memories or emotions in a flash. You want to start a new diet. This triggers the belief that you can and will be your best self a year from now. Or it will trigger that you've never succeeded so don't try.

Consider the crab. One crab in a bucket might try to scale the side and escape. But a bucketful of crabs changes everything. One crab tries to scale the side and another crab will invariably pull the adventurous crab back down. Eventually, all the crabs just stay in the bucket and don't try to escape.

But your brain is the command center, you are in command, and you can decide if a program upgrade is needed. New grooves. A new plan to get out of the bucket.

The brain houses the triggers, but it also supplies the willpower to make the changes. It's just an excuse if you blame lack of willpower for not accomplishing something.

Excuses. Rationalizations. To make you feel better, but it's not the truth. Repeated thinking like this, though, is a trigger to not try. It's just old programming.

If you combine new awareness of what triggers you with new information about willpower, you can reprogram your brain power. You might amaze yourself as you tackle old beliefs and new goals.

Willpower

Willpower isn't just gritting your teeth and willing yourself to do the thing you should do but don't want to. It's a brain function, fueled by glucose.

Sleep resets your willpower. You wake up with your full dose of willpower every day. We all do. We start fresh every day.

Willpower allows us to control an initial impulse or postpone instant gratification in order to achieve the desired result.

We don't think of willpower as our decision-making power. Most people think it's some superpower you pull out to stop you from doing something wrong.

In the moment we might whip out our excuses ("It's too hard" or "It takes too long.") We exercise willpower by making a better decision to accomplish our goal.

All decisions are drawn from your daily supply. If you've made a lot of decisions throughout the day, you'll find yourself with decision fatigue in the evening. That's what you've been calling lack of willpower.

Yes, it can be difficult to resist temptation. It's easier to grab a bag of chips. And reaching for those chips just triggered a fond memory of couch and tv time.

If you don't know what foods you're going to eat, then the decision-making process becomes harder. Especially at night.

If you want to control your diabetes, lose weight, and eat well, you need to start with a plan.

With depleted willpower, people make rash decisions and don't process information well. That's why so many infomercials play late at night. Viewers are far more likely to buy at 2 am than at 2 pm.

It's easy to start the day with a To Do list and just pick all the easy tasks first. It looks like more has been accomplished because there are more boxes checked off.

This depletes a lot of willpower on small decisions. Prioritizing tasks and working on the highest payoff task will bring greater benefit, both in what gets done and in maintaining more willpower.

Experienced project planners focus on doing the highest priority tasks first. They may not consciously realize that it's simply a smart willpower decision.

If you have multiple projects going at once, pick the most important and focus there first. Of course, you can accomplish others at the same time. Just know your peak times for intense projects vs. time to work on lesser ones.

Pick your battles. Know your limits. If you get frustrated around certain people, avoid them whenever possible. Some families agree to limit how long they will be at extended family functions.

Choose alert, high willpower times for meetings where tensions might run high. Don't confront people at night when you both have decision fatigue.

If you find yourself saying you just don't have the willpower to continue healthy eating, it's probably because you're making too many decisions at the wrong time of day. You can plan at night, but you need adequate sleep and then you can execute your plan when your willpower has been replenished.

Try preparing foods ahead, like veggie snacks. Then you're less likely to lose the willpower battle when hungry. A shopping list means less decision making in the store. That tempting pastry display is less likely to trigger bad choices.

Set a specific time for exercise. You won't have to decide every day if, when, or what you need to do. You know. Just go do it.

Even though you start the day with the same amount of willpower, every decision, large or small, depletes your supply throughout the day.

So, what are all these decisions? Get up or hit the snooze button, what to wear, what to eat for breakfast, helping other family members before heading to work, check on traffic, decide what route to drive. Do you stop for donuts and coffee, or should you skip it? And all before you even get to work to start that part of your day.

If you are sleep deprived, you may have lower willpower reserves at the beginning of the day. Remember, willpower is restored during sleep.

You're also more susceptible to illness, like colds or flu, when decision fatigue is high. Whether or not you recognize it at the time, your stamina is low.

The good news is you can supercharge your willpower.

Actions can be fueled by emotions. Actions with willpower are fueled by thought. Your head must be in charge to override emotional impulses. I'm sure you've heard the saying, "Act your way into a feeling." I've had to repeat that to myself many times when I simply don't feel like doing what I know I should do.

You can also have a predetermined rule that in certain temptations you will wait a while before deciding. It may be that this is an emotion-driven decision that vaporizes when you wait. This works well for me when I see something unexpected that screams "buy me."

Know your "why," and visualize yourself having attained your goal. Create a vision board to remind you daily of your goals. Develop a routine for when and where you'll do certain repetitive tasks. This subconsciously strengthens your resolve (willpower) by removing some of the temptations and decisions.

Willpower can be strengthened by exercise. Have you ever noticed that after a brisk walk or an intense workout, you are recharged and can take on more decisions? The exercise refuels your willpower reserves.

You can reduce stress with yoga, tai chi, meditation or prayer.

One decision that will help you minimize decision fatigue is making a commitment to reach a specific goal, such as becoming healthy.

> Commitment is doing what you said you would do long after the feeling in which you said it has left you.

Being aware of these facts help with your choices, reduces stress triggers, and doesn't over-deplete your willpower. Prioritize your health goals, make them clear and know when you need to do what.

Think about how you can use triggers and willpower in your favor by reviewing the information about hype and sabotage.

17

Who's in Charge?

Since 1950, more than 600,000 packaged and processed foods have been introduced into the marketplace. Eighty percent of them are full of sugar, often tablespoons and tablespoons, hidden and disguised by all sorts of names.

Processed foods hide behind good marketing and labeling. But processed foods are not healthy foods. They are chemically treated and not what we were intended to eat to keep our brain and body functioning well. Their ingredients can cause weight gain. What we call junk food is so over-processed that it isn't really food—it's just junk.

Grain products are stripped of their natural nutrients and then fortified to placate consumers who expect nutrition as well as good flavor or ease of preparation.

Contaminants have become a growing issue with food recalls. One issue, E. coli, affects a growing number of people, even causing death.

For the past 40 years, over 300 scientists at the Monell Chemical Senses Center in Philadelphia have explored why we love food as we do. The food industry is very involved in their research.

Taxpayers fund about half of the multi-million-dollar budget, with the rest coming from the food and tobacco industries. Although they claim to be impartial with their studies, Monell still focuses on large amounts of research for the food industry. This aids in producing highly processed foods that keep the customer coming back for more.

The major food companies want to train consumers on how and what to eat. That should be a red flag.

With over 300 million people in the United States, the Department of Agriculture (USDA) is charged with overseeing and protecting the people from themselves. But there are about 300 companies in a $1 trillion industry of food manufacturing, many with active lobby groups. The USDA feels obligated to work with and nurture this group. Do you see the disconnect? The contradictions?

We are the ones who must be proactive in reading labels, understanding ingredients and how much sugar, fat, and salt they contain. Many ingredients are non-essential to humans but essential to the food manufacturers in getting high sales and shelf life for their products.

Hand-wringing stories of how diabetes has become not just an epidemic, but a pandemic (which means worldwide), act as if there must be a bad gene or some other ancient factor involved.

Statements that it's inherited and unavoidable are coupled with gloomy statements that you need the drugs they prescribe, or you'll die even sooner. Myths grew rapidly.

Scientists, doctors, and government agencies skip over the changes that occurred in the 1900s. It's as if they can't figure out the correlation between farming changes and food industry events that began after the depression era of the '30s, World War II in the '40s, and a booming economy in the '50s.

Enter industrialization of the food industry and things like farm subsidies and lobby groups. Some ideas were good on the surface but lacked the foresight to anticipate negative side effects.

It's a hot topic, deluged with information all over the board. It's total confusion about what to safely eat.

With the food industry sabotaging you, struggling with overcoming diabetes and weight loss isn't totally your fault.

> Today, by the time the average child in a developed country turns 8 years old, they've had more sugar in their lives than the average person did in their entire lifetime just one century ago. —PreventDisease.com

Proactive steps you can take

- Cut out all soft drinks and fruit juices.
- Eliminate all "Fast Food"
- Eat freshly prepared food, not convenient imitation food.

- Reduce or eliminate the amount of meat you eat.
- Increase the amount of fiber in your diet.
- Drink no more than 4 glasses of red wine a week.
- Snack on fresh fruit and nuts instead of cookies and candy. Be cautious with the nut, seeds, and dried fruit combos. There's a lot of sugar in dried fruit.
- Hunger may really be thirst. Resolve it with water, preferably room temperature with lemon, lime or other fruit slices added.
- When eating out, order two or three sides of vegetables and skip the bread and pasta, which are proven to pack on the pounds and contribute to diabetes.

18

What's Best: Food Do's and Don'ts

"Let food be thy medicine,
and medicine be thy food."
—HIPPOCRATES,
THE ANCIENT GREEK PHYSICIAN

- Eat more veggies
- Eliminate sugar and cut down on carbs
- Eat more whole foods

You didn't get to this diagnosis overnight. You undoubtedly ate foods that haven't served you well. However, if you choose well now, and stick with it, you should be able to master your numbers and extend your life. When the foods you take in are healthy choices, your body is going to function better, plus extra body weight should melt away.

There are many diet plans focused on diabetes. You can adopt one of them or learn what foods are best at controlling your sugar levels and what foods to avoid, then create your own eating plan. My book *Diabetes Diet Options* discusses seven different diets. Whatever you choose, it doesn't have to be boring or overly restrictive.

Choose whole foods for their nutritional value, especially since they will contain a variety of nutrients.

Being consistent and having variety in your diet at the same time is possible!

The consistency comes with specific meal times and the serving sizes. The variety refers to trying as many new foods or new combinations as you can. You have a lot of room for flexibility.

Just because you have diabetes doesn't mean you can't be adventurous and try something new. Just do it at regular meal times and within the recommended portion sizes. The stronger your why, the better your results.

Unfortunately, much of our foods are over-processed and insufficient, so supplements are advisable. Choose fresh whole vegetables and fruits. Fruit juices lose their fiber value and end up being mostly sugary calories.

Diet Fads

Diet fads come and go. Some are stranger than others, some even harmful. Some are simple-to-do, but they don't really provide health benefits.

Smoothies can be healthy – but not always

Many smoothies are healthy, and they're a good way to get a lot of veggies or fruits and nutrients into your system. Green veggie smoothies provide nutrition and an easy way to consume vegetables, but many people assume they won't like the taste and simply won't even try them. They think it's too hard to drink it while holding their nose.

So they add sugar loaded yogurt or other flavor cover-ups that add unnecessary calories to the greens. Others just aim to taste sweet, and they give a false belief that you are eating healthy.

Some people claim they don't like vegetables and prefer fruits. So for them, they make daily fruit smoothies, some with peanut butter or sweetened yogurt. Do you have any idea how many calories those fruit smoothies have, to say nothing of the sugar and high glycemic count? This is serious if you have prediabetes or type 2.

Have you heard about this fad diet?

Just eat one food, all day, every day, for an extended number of days. The theory here is you'll get so sick of it after three or four days that you'll just eat less and less, and that's how you lose weight.

It doesn't matter if it's steak, peanut butter, milkshakes, or carrots. And if you choose the milkshakes and get sick of it after four days, you're most likely just going to quit. So, four days of high calorie, insulin-shocking, non-nutrition? It'll probably set you back several more pounds and damage your organs even more. Sure, that sounds like a lot of fun.

Calorie source matters

Yes, there is a Twinkie diet. 200 Twinkie calories provide no nutrition and are quickly converted to fat. They're sugar and refined carbs.

200 calories from a pile of veggies, salad or a lean steak provide healthy nutrients with little or no fat added to your body.

If you eat only Twinkies, let's say 900 calories for the entire day, it will be quickly converted to belly fat. At 900 calories you will lose some weight to start out, but at what cost? Your health will suffer because of lack of nutrients.

You'll feel full after the salad or steak, but not the Twinkie, so you're probably going to eat more than the 900 calories in our example. It's a bad plan for a non-diabetic, and a horrible one for a diabetic.

Cute food names don't build cute bodies. But they build large bank accounts for the companies that make up the names.

Antioxidants and Vitamins

Many studies in recent years have proven that antioxidants help prevent diabetic complications, especially neuropathy and retinopathy. Most people know we need them, but questions remain, like how much and which ones.

Antioxidant experts call diabetes a "free radical disease." People with diabetes use up their antioxidant stores more quickly, so their requirements are significantly higher. This is because diabetes creates more free radicals, and free radicals use up the vitamins, therefore, you need more.

Vitamins are also flushed through a diabetic's body at an alarming rate. Make sure you take proper dosages of necessary vitamins to give your body the best possible chance for absorbing what you need.

Be sure to take a good multivitamin. Consider the special diabetic packs since you simply aren't going to get enough through food alone. This may be true for all of us with the highly processed foods we eat, but it's much more so for the diabetic.

One of the often overlooked but very important vitamins is Vitamin D, known as the sunshine vitamin. It improves insulin sensitivity by up to 60%, according to extensive research. Those are better numbers than the diabetic drug metformin.

It also has been shown to lessen complications of cardiovascular disease. Some foods high in Vitamin D include liver (I know, everyone's favorite), wild salmon, shrimp, cod, eggs, and milk. Also add red, yellow and orange fruits and vegetables and dark green leafy vegetables.

Ask your physician to check your Vitamin D. It's sometimes overlooked in the typical vitamin packs, so you'll want to know if you need extra supplements.

Water

Common belief teaches you should drink up to half your body weight of water in ounces, daily. Others teach 48-64 oz daily. The reality is that typical tap water just flushes vitamins and minerals from your body. Add juice from a fresh lemon to aid in digestion. Add ¼ tsp of unrefined sea salt per quart of water to help get water into the cells. Best practice: just drink when thirsty, especially quality mineral water.

A glass of water first thing in the morning on an empty stomach plumps your cells and helps prepare you for the day ahead.

With diabetes, only some cells get survival rations of water. Continuous dehydration can, in time, cause massive damage to the blood vessels throughout the body. It can cause or contribute to the eventual loss of toes, feet, and legs from gangrene, as well as eye damage and even blindness.

Alcohol

In moderation of course. If you drink alcohol, choose red wine. The skin of red grapes is a rich source of red wine's natural compound resveratrol. This may help diabetics regulate their blood sugar, according to recent research published in the journal *Nutrition.*

Drink only four glasses a week maximum, preferably less. And no, I don't mean it's ok to use the overly large novelty glasses.

Many doctors or studies indicate it's okay to drink one-to-two glasses of red wine a day, but when you also figure in the reaction it has on your brain and sleep cycle, the recommendation goes to four glasses per week.

White wine is next best, but it has a slightly higher sugar count and doesn't have the resveratrol benefit. What about beer and margaritas? Not so much. Did you know a single 12 oz margarita has over 1100 calories and a high concentration of sugar? If you do have a beer or margarita, be sure it's balanced with other healthy foods (sorry, not nachos or cheese fries) and only one on planned occasions.

Drinking alcohol to excess can contribute to people becoming diabetic. Prediabetics should be aware of this. Serious consumption reduces the body's sensitivity to insulin, which can trigger type 2 diabetic issues. Drinking contributes to pancreas issues. Alcoholic beverages contain a massive quantity of calories. Drinking contributes not only to the beer belly but also diabetic issues.

Fiber

The role of fiber in healthy diets is very important. It aids in digestion and keeps your colon and other organs healthy and functioning properly. It's also something that should be a large part of any diabetic's diet. You will reap many benefits by including fiber in your diet. If you're prediabetic, it can assist in delaying or avoiding a diagnosis of diabetes. If you're already diabetic, it can help keep your blood glucose under control.

Fiber will keep you feeling fuller longer. It slows the conversion of carbohydrates in your body which in turn can keep your blood sugar stable. The type of fiber needed to gain these benefits is soluble fiber (dissolves in water) such as the fiber in vegetables.

A serving of broccoli will fill you up (high satiety level) but an entire bag of potato chips will not notify your brain that you are full. So, you keep eating.

Some sources of soluble fiber include:

- Sprouted or whole grain products instead of white flour, breads, and cereals
- Vegetables and some fresh fruits. Don't choose the processed version or drink them in liquid form (eliminates the fiber but keeps the sugar)
- Beans: use dried beans in your favorite recipes like chili for a wholesome, high-fiber meal

To ensure that you are getting the most benefit from eating an increased amount of fiber, be sure to drink 48-64 oz. of water daily (that's three-to-four 16-ounce water bottles). You need to stay hydrated for fiber to work properly. If this amount of water seems like "too much" right now, then drink as much as possible, consistently working toward 48- 64-ounces daily.

Carbs

Overconsumption of carbs is the primary driving factor for insulin resistance and type 2 diabetes.

By eating good carbohydrate choices and lean meats you will lower the insulin requirements for your body. All foods you eat affect your blood sugars, and it affects how your cells can accept the increased glucose. Poor dietary choices can have serious long-term effects on your body and its organs.

Unfortunately, the dietary establishment has unwisely been praising the virtues of carbohydrates while warning you to avoid fats. But anyone who bought into the high-carb, low-fat diets has likely struggled with their weight and health, wondering what they're doing wrong.

The truth of the matter is that a diet high in grain carbs (as opposed to vegetables) and low in fat may be dangerous to your health, and if you want to shed excess weight and improve your health, the opposite diet is what you're looking for!

In other words, when you eat too much bread, pasta, and any other grain products, you're essentially sending a hormonal message, via insulin, to your body that says "store fat."

Additionally, increased insulin levels also

- Make it virtually impossible for you to use your own stored body fat for energy
- Suppress two important hormones: glucagon and growth hormone. Glucagon 35 promotes the burning of fat and sugar. Growth hormone is used for muscle development and building new muscle mass.
- Increases hunger: As blood sugar increases following a carbohydrate meal, insulin rises with the eventual result of lower blood sugar. This results in hunger, often only a couple of hours (or less) after the meal.

So, all in all, the excess carbohydrates in your diet not only make you fat, they make sure you stay fat. Cravings, usually for sweets, frequently result in snacking on more carbohydrates. Not eating can make you feel ravenous, shaky, moody and ready to crash.

If the problem is chronic, you'll never get rid of that stored fat, and your energy and overall health is adversely affected.

Carbohydrates to Avoid:

- High fructose corn syrup
- Sugar
- Processed grains
- White flour

Carbohydrates that are OK

- Vegetables, especially colorful ones. No restrictions
- Fruits, berries, and cherries—fresh, organic is best
- If not on keto—whole intact grains like brown or black rice, quinoa, buckwheat and bulgur
- Beans but not the ones with added sugars (you'd be surprised where that's hiding out)
- Proteins that are ok
- Wild Caught fish, salmon, black cod sardines, arctic char
- Omega 3 enriched eggs
- Organic dairy like unsweetened plain yogurt and hard cheeses in small amounts

Herbs and Spices

All are ok. Many healthy recipes include these. Use in detox, others are flavor and nutrient providers. They've been used for centuries for healing. Some examples:

- turmeric
- ginger
- cloves
- cumin
- paprika
- sage
- rosemary
- cayenne
- cinnamon
- garlic

Protein

Much the same as fiber, eating quality protein with your snacks and meals can have a positive effect on your blood sugar levels. By combining protein and good carbohydrates you will slow the digestion of the carbohydrates in your body. This will prevent your blood sugar from spiking.

Don't eat more protein than is recommended in one meal. Doing so can lead to other problems down the road. Health experts recommend 4-6 oz. of protein as a serving.

Skipping protein in your diet is not wise. For vegetarians or diabetics who usually don't eat a lot of protein, it's important to find a source that can be consumed on a regular basis, such as nuts and seeds, beans, fish, and powdered protein that can be added to shakes.

Turkey, fish, and cheese have the highest protein-to-calorie ratio. Cottage cheese and low-fat mozzarella are the cheeses with the highest protein.

Proteins to Avoid

- Factory farmed beef. Cattle are fed mostly corn, are heavily medicated, unhealthy animals.
- Avoid all pork
- Factory farmed poultry and eggs

Proteins that are OK

- Wild caught salmon, black cod, sardines, arctic char
- Omega 3 enriched eggs
- Beans (see carb notes)
- Organic dairy such as unsweetened plain yogurt, cottage cheese and hard cheeses in small amounts

Vegetables and Fruits

Scientific research overwhelmingly tells us that the single most important thing we can do for our health is to eat more vegetables and fruits. In fact, it is about the only thing that every nutritional philosophy agrees upon.

Life expectancy would grow by leaps and bounds if green vegetables smelled as good as bacon.

Plant foods contain a rich combination of blood-sugar-balancing, anti-inflammatory, detoxifying compounds called phytonutrients.

Inflammation has been linked to most of the diseases of aging, including heart attacks, diabetes, cancer, and dementia. In fact, being overweight is a chronic inflammatory state. Vegetables and fruits contain nature's most powerful anti-inflammatories.

Plant foods are the main source of vitamins and minerals in your diet. These vitamins and minerals run every chemical reaction in your body.

Seek out these nutrients

- Omega 3 (fish, natural supplements)
- Choline (found in eggs)
- Creatine
- CoEnzyme Q10
- Amino acids (protein)
- Vitamin B Complex
- Vitamin C
- Vitamin D (sunshine is a useful source of this too!)
- Lutein
- Magnesium
- Zinc

Food Ideas from Breakfast to Bedtime

- Burrito - scrambled eggs, onions, peppers, black beans, salsa, cheese, whole grain tortilla
- Cottage cheese and fresh fruit
- Power smoothie (not the sugary fruit smoothies)
- Hard boiled eggs and cheese
- Turkey or chicken layered on sprouted whole grain bread, tomato, avocado
- Lean chicken, turkey sausage, wild caught salmon
- Plain yogurt with fresh blueberries
- Range free eggs, omega 3 fortified
- Veggie scramble, black beans, and cheese
- Pair fruits with nuts, cheeses
- Nuts, seeds. Best nuts are almonds and walnuts
- Healing vegetables: 3–5 servings per day, raw veggies best
- Salads—dark greens like Romaine better than iceberg
- Lightly steamed veggies (or microwave)
- Raw veggie snacks
- Mashed cauliflower as a potato substitute
- Cauliflower pizzas (great taste, usually gluten-free, and much lower calories)
- Steamed veggies, brown rice, chicken or salmon
- Deep sea, cold water fish (2-3 times/week)
- Wild Pacific salmon (Atlantic salmon is often really farmed and not healthy)

- Tuna, halibut. rainbow trout, scallops
- Grass fed, high-quality meats
- Buffalo (bison) – grass fed and no antibiotics so it's actually better than beef
- French cheeses or American only from grass-fed cows
- Thin turkey slice with veggies – not processed turkey
- Celery sticks with cream cheese or peanut butter
- Veggies and cheese (not processed)
- Dips from yogurt and diced cucumbers, etc. with veggie sticks
- Eat salads, veggies, beans, salmon, hard boiled eggs
- 64 oz of water daily
- Sparkling water
- Add fruit or veggie slices to a pitcher of water (encourages drinking more)
- Water with fresh lemons first thing in the morning -wakes up the cells, fights dehydration
- 1/4 unsweetened pomegranate or blueberry juice to 3/4 sparkling water
- Don't use powdered packaged flavorings
- Stevia-sweetened Soda Stream mixes (moderate use)
- Coffee - black, regular or decaf
- Tea (green, black, red)
- Hearty non-GMO whole grains
- Ezekiel bread, sprouted grain

- Unsweetened homemade granola
- Add fruits, cinnamon
- Whole grain pasta (Racconto brand)
- Rye, barley, quinoa

This list is not inclusive, but it will give you a starting point about healthy foods and suggested combinations. I've added comments for some items. With fish, be sure to select wild caught and not farmed fish. Tilapia is a common, inexpensive fish option but should be avoided. It's farmed, has compromised nutrition, low omega-3 and high omega 6, and has been shown to contribute to inflammation.

Focus on These Foods

Proteins/4oz	**Cal**	**Vegetables/4oz**	**Cal**	**Fruits**	**Cal**
Bass	140	Arugula	7	Apple 1 med	95
Beef	247	Asparagus	5	Apricots	34
Buffalo	229	Beet Greens	6	Blackberries, ½ c	31
Chicken	219	Bell peppers	6	Blueberries ½ c	42
Cod	119	Broccoli	10	Cherries ½ c	49
Cottage Cheese	96	Brussel sprouts	12	½ grapefruit	41
Crab	126	Cabbage	7	Lemon 1 oz.	8
Elk	165	Cauliflower	7	Orange 1med	62
Flounder/Sole	132	Celery	4	½ pear	52
Grouper	133	Chard	5	½ peach	34
Haddock	127	Cucumbers	4	Plum, 2	60
Halibut	128	Endive/escarole	5	Strawberries oz.	9
Lobster	131	Fennel	9	Tomatoes oz.	5
Mahi Mahi	140	Green beans	9		
Perch	132	Hearts of Palm	8	Red wine 4oz.	96
Roughy	119	Kale	14	White wine 4oz.	96
Wild-caught salmon*	161	Lettuce (all)	4		
Scallops	128	Mushrooms (all)	8	Glass of wine is ok, but Margaritas have too much sugar.	
Shrimp	131	Onion	12		
Tuna	154	Radishes	5		
Turkey	212	Spinach	7	**Healthy oils**	
Veal	224	Tomatoes oz.	5	Avocado oil	
Venison	168	Watercress	8	Coconut oil	
Whole Egg	55	Zucchini	6	Extra Virgin Olive Oil	

* Wild-caught salmon has 1/2 the calories and saturated fat of farmed salmon. Always coosse the wild-caught slamon.

Enjoy lots of veggies, eat fruits selectively as they have more natural sugar. Eliminate added sugars, eat moderate amouts of carbs (veggies have good carbs), eat only healthy fats and oil. Avoid processed foods.

19

What About a Detox?

Even if the idea of detoxing doesn't sound like much fun, you should check out these very real benefits, especially if you want to jumpstart better health.

Imagine a dry sponge being dripped on. Eventually, it will become saturated and overflow with whatever was dripping on it, either good or bad. It's the old techno rule: Garbage In, Garbage Out.

When it comes to what we put into our bodies, it's ideal to start eating healthy at a young age to prevent eventual breakdown. Unfortunately, most of us are way past that "young age." We didn't realize that the "garbage in" doesn't show up as "garbage out" for many years. It's invisibly compounding on the inside.

With all the toxins that surround us daily, it's important to consciously detox our bodies. This is important for everyone, whether or not you are prediabetic or type 2. You can jump-start cleansing your system to regain your best health.

Detoxification entails purifying the blood. It does this chiefly by getting rid of impurities from the blood in the liver, where toxins are refined for excretion. The body likewise eliminates toxins through the kidneys, bowels, lungs, lymph, and skin. When this system is compromised, impurities are not properly filtrated and every cell in the body is adversely affected.

You are only fasting from foods that harm you.

If a detox will help you jumpstart healthy eating or even weight loss, then you should consider doing it. It should help your body's natural cleansing process by:

1) Giving the organs a rest with modified fasting
2) Getting the liver to push toxins from the body
3) Raising elimination through the bowels, kidneys, and skin
4) Improving the circulation of the blood
5) Refueling the body with sound nutrients

Eliminate foods that cause toxicity in the first place. Some toxins are released through perspiration. If you have access to a sauna, use it to flush toxins out of the body.

During a detox, eliminate alcohol, coffee, tobacco, sugars and concentrated fats which act as toxins in the system. Increase the amount of water that you drink to help flush the toxins. You aren't doing a complete food-fast. You are only fasting from foods that harm you.

Minimize the use of chemical-based house cleaners and personal healthcare products and replace with organic alternatives. This is wise with or without a detox. Most antiperspirants, for example, add aluminum, which is toxic. Products that add fragrance are adding toxins into your body. The term "fragrance" includes about a thousand different chemical product options. You won't know which ones since government regulations only require the product label to list the word "fragrance."

Length of detoxing varies but is usually 3-5 days. Since you have diabetes to consider, you might think in terms of 2-3 days, or whatever your doctor deems safe.

Check with your medical professional for what you specifically can do. You still need to consume the proper nutrients to keep your blood sugar in the proper range. If you're up for it and your doctor agrees, try veggie smoothies so you maintain a liquid type diet for a couple of days. This lets your systems rest, but you still get the nutrients you need.

You should feel so much better with the liquid version or small intentional meals. Your numbers might dip into the lower range because your body doesn't need as much of the medications you are taking. Again, be sure you are working with your doctor and not self-diagnosing when it comes to your meds.

Continue to eat clean and healthy after detoxing, which should keep your glucose levels in a proper range. If they dip lower, it could indicate you don't need as much medication. Your doctor may even start weaning you off the meds.

There are safe detox plans such as veggie juices and some clear fruit juices, like apple and cranberry juice. Be cautious with fruit juices as they are much higher in sugar than vegetables, but they do let your digestive system rest. Avoid orange juice during a fast, since it is so high in sugar. If you purchase detox drinks, make sure they're organic, cold pressed and not from concentrate.

After a detox program, you should be able to keep your body toxin free through diet, supplements and lifestyle changes which help you reach an ideal weight and reboot your health.

I believe the importance of detoxing is in what you don't eat: no sugar, flour, rice, potatoes, and none of the carbs that you're detoxing. If you suspect allergies, then you'll want to eliminate those possible offenders as well.

Once detoxed, you can start adding some eliminated foods back into your diet, but not all at once. If something eliminated is a toxic food for you, you'll want to know what it is without masking it with everything else.

Mental Detox

We've talked about how the myths, excuses and sabotage have hijacked our thinking about our health and whether we can overcome lifestyle diseases or not. We've already cracked open the limiting beliefs.

So, while we take better care of our bodies, what about our thoughts? What most of us *don't* think about is *what* we think about.

When we change our beliefs on the inside, we transform the results we see on the outside.

Unconsciously we go about dealing with daily tasks, situations, traffic, long lines, slow internet, and other people. Years ago, I heard motivational speaker Connie Podesta start her talk with *"Life would be great if it weren't for other people."* Humorous and true enough, but not possible.

So, once aware, how do we detox our minds, our thoughts, and feelings? Entire volumes are written about how to do this. I can only offer some suggestions to get you started.

How about aiming to collapse the limiting beliefs you've absorbed? Or detox life situations at the same time you detox your body? What thoughts and feelings come bubbling up right now?

To mentally detox, allow yourself to become aware of thoughts that have an emotional trigger, make you angry, or disappointed. Is there something you think is holding you back?

As I mentioned in the chapter on the brain, stress can lead to disease, and repeated focus on things that are stressful to you will eventually damage your health and your spirit. So, a mental detox and a body detox give you a double boost up.

Think about the people you're repeatedly around. If some are negative family members or co-workers, you may need to limit the time you're together or just be mindful with your thoughts during time together. Realizing that angry situations can't force you to become angry makes it easier to keep your cool. I don't mean excusing the actions of others, but rather, not allowing them to derail you.

Les Brown, now a well-known speaker, knew from personal experience that harsh words can demoralize the listener. But a wise teacher turned his life around when he told him, *"Don't let someone else's opinion of you become your reality."*

Become aware and release negative thoughts. Replace them with gratitude thoughts. A negative heart and a grateful heart can't co-exist. The heart and brain constantly communicate through a complex network of cells, and surprisingly most messages go from your heart to your brain. So, your emotions can bully your thoughts.

If your self-talk tells you that you're (insert negative talk) then you need to change that to "I deserve to be healthy" or whatever is the positive version of what you tell yourself. Keep saying it so your emotions pick up on your tremendous value.

You can focus on mental detoxing at specific times, or just pay attention to your thoughts throughout the day. As you purposefully choose to release stressful thoughts or self-doubt, you will experience more peace and less anxiety. Your reaction can even unconsciously defuse the other person's attitude as well. Not always, but sometimes.

Yoga and quieting the mind through prayer or meditation are simple and effective ways to remedy tension. It recharges your physical and mental powers to overcome the inevitable tension life will bring. Even 5 minutes daily will benefit you.

It might be sitting silently for 5-10 minutes and not some fancy ritual. Think about your goals and how good you'll feel to accomplish them. Focus on your breathing, with purposeful, slow deep breaths. This will calm your heart and, in turn, will calm your mind.

The body is a complex but integrated machine. When you eat harmful foods, hold negative emotions like fear, self-doubt, anger or unforgiveness, or focus on stressful thoughts, your brain is affected and even shrinks. Brain fog can set in. It can be reversed by releasing negative emotions, even if only for a few minutes at a time.

There's a story of a businessman who arrived home after work, parked in the driveway, and on the way into the house placed an imaginary bundle on a tree branch. In the morning he reversed the process. A neighbor observed him do this several times, and one morning asked him about it. He smiled and replied, *"I'm leaving my work problems outside. I pick them back up if I need to think about a solution on the way to work the next day."*

No one can force you to think a certain way. But when others tell us lies or hurtful things, it's very hard to ignore until we know the truth. A conscious mental detox gives you a chance to show that you get to be the commander of your emotions and thoughts. Choose wisely, live long and prosper. And celebrate!

20

Exercise

An early morning walk is a blessing
for the whole day.
—HENRY DAVID THOREAU

One of the most undemanding and workable ways to regulate blood sugar, eliminate the dangers of cardiovascular disease, and perk up health and welfare and increase willpower reserves is exercise. Any exercise is better than none.

Combine healthy eating with regular exercise. This is good for your insulin requirements and blood glucose levels. By incorporating exercise into your daily routine, you can give your body's metabolism a boost and help it process the foods you're eating.

We live in an inactive world where many jobs are managed from an ergonomic chair in front of a computer. Electronic games and social media keep people tied to computers and mobile devices.

Exercise can come last in your thoughts and your day's event planning.

For about two-thirds of the population, the idea of exercise is just that: an idea. It feels overwhelming. Even when they make a resolution to exercise, it rarely lasts more than six weeks.

When you think of exercise, think movement. That seems less threatening. It's never too late to get moving, and it's one of the easiest ways to start controlling your diabetes. It also boosts willpower reserves which can come in handy in resisting poor choice foods.

Movement can improve insulin sensitivity, lower the risk of heart disease, and promote weight loss.

Getting Started

The first thing to do as you decide on an exercise program is to consult with your health care provider. If you have cardiac risk factors, the health care provider may want to perform a stress test to establish a safe level of exercise for you.

Certain diabetic complications will also dictate what type of exercise program you can take on. Activities like weightlifting, jogging, or high-impact aerobics can possibly pose a risk for people with diabetic retinopathy due to the risk for further blood vessel damage and possible retinal detachment.

If you are already active in sports or work out regularly, it will still benefit you to discuss your regular routine with your doctor.

If you're feeling out of shape, perhaps you can do a little more than whatever you're currently doing.

Start slowly, like walking for 10-15 minutes 3-4 times a week. If you're extremely overweight and out of shape, you may need to start with a walk to the mailbox and back. Seriously. Your first exercise might be pushing away from the table.

There are exercise programs like yoga and tai chi that are effective and easy to start if you're not used to any exercise. There's even a tai chi program sitting down! You can Google it.

Your exercise routine can be as simple as a brisk nightly neighborhood walk. If you haven't been very active before now, start slowly and work your way up. Walk the dog or get out in the yard and rake leaves. Take the stairs instead of the elevator. Park in the back of the lot and walk. Every little bit works. In fact, it helps a lot.

As little as 15 to 30 minutes of heart-pumping exercise can make a big difference in your blood glucose control and help prevent developing diabetic complications. Ramp it up as you get used to the routine and your health care provider says it's ok.

You don't have to invest in costly health club memberships, or the most up-to-date health device to start pumping out the fat. What you need is the willingness and the determination to start exercising to achieve a healthier lifestyle.

21

Taking Control

Your lifestyle – how you live, eat, emote, and think – determines your health. To prevent disease, you may have to change how you live.
—BRIAN CARTER, BUSINESS CONSULTANT

Sometimes you're doing exactly what you need to do, and you get impressive results. Then a monkey wrench gets thrown in and you get to begin again. From personal experience, it can sneak up on you and takes effort to recover what you've messed up.

We did some renovating. Our new hardwood floors required ripping up the kitchen tile. It was a mess. So, we went out for lunch and dinner. Every day. We kept eating out for about 2 months after the floors were finished.

We usually selected the best of the worst from the menu, whether sandwiches for lunch or full dinners. On occasion, it probably wouldn't have been such an impact.

We were getting food that we had no control over. We had processed foods and carbs out of control. How the kitchens prepared the meals was unknown. It spoiled the best of our intentions to the tune of about 10-15 pounds gained. Each.

There were things we could have done differently to save the weight gains. But we didn't. We didn't realize how quickly we could pile on the pounds. Because the blood glucose numbers remained good, we rationalized that eating out that much could be okay. Nope.

So, we faced the facts. We restarted our weight loss routine with a much better understanding of why eating out can be so dangerous.

We knew what to do, so why didn't we do it? It was easy to do and easy not to do. Excuses, decision fatigue, we all go there from time to time.

Any day you mess up is an opportunity to start again. Make a mental note of why you gave in to temptation. This will help you next time temptation shows up.

Ask yourself

- What time of day did it happen?
- What else was going on?
- Were you overtired?

- Were you having to make a lot of decisions during the day?
- Were you on emotional overload?
- Did something stressful happen that took you off course?

Or if you're like me, a "let's do lunch" opportunity with someone you enjoy having face-to-face time with can be the trigger to eat out instead of at home. It might be one temptation too many as you look at the menu. I usually choose a salad with balsamic dressing on the side, but not always. We can rationalize anything when our resolve is weakened. Remember decision fatigue?

The Hardest Part IS Getting Started

A man was driving through a small town and stopped at a hardware store. Two men were rocking on a porch outside of the store. There was a hound dog off to the side, howling in pain every couple of minutes.

The traveler asked why the dog was howling.

"He's sitting on a nail poking through the board."

"Why doesn't he move?"

"It doesn't hurt enough."

Does your nail hurt enough? That's what it will take to overcome your diabetes. It's a lifelong choice, it will take effort and some struggles. There may be times when you want to go back to the old ways that got you to your diagnosis. This is when your commitment will be important.

I'm assuming you're already determined and now is your time to turn things around. I applaud you!

Most of the benefits of sleep, exercise, and diet come from just doing the basics. First, decide what you want to accomplish, then act immediately.

You will be in control because no one else can accomplish this for you. Control is different from doing it all by yourself, however.

It's important to know what you can control, and what you can't. You can control your actions, and how consistently you work toward your goals. You can't control the things added to food, nor the amount of sabotage mentioned earlier, nor the quality of the products on the market. It's best if you have a family member, friend or coach encouraging you and holding you accountable. You aren't in control of what they say, but you can control your reaction to them. Positive reaction = good results.

1. Decide to do this now. It's the only time you can control. The past is over. Forgive yourself for past mistakes as needed and move on to now. You aren't in the future yet, so all you have is NOW.

2. Get a full blood workup, not just of your A1C and blood glucose and blood pressure. Ask to have the doctor check inflammation markers, vitamin D, hormones, how your vital organs are doing, and whatever you and your doctor think advisable. If you get a solid baseline of where your body is NOW, you will have a way of evaluating how well you're progressing toward rebooting your health.

3. Go through your pantry and refrigerator. Remove all the foods that will derail you. If you have other family members who want foods that you can't have, try separating your foods from theirs to make cheating less tempting. Discuss your needs with them and work together for success.

4. Create a meal plan that you can live with. Use the guidelines in the chapter, *What's Best: Food Do's and Don'ts.* Make it as simple as you can to start. Agree to give it at least a 30-day trial, then I hope you'll agree to another two months to establish new habits.

5. Talk out loud about your plans. This can be with family and friends, or just to yourself. When you talk out loud, your brain hears what you say, and it carves new grooves in your brain. Be sure you speak positive affirmations. Your new groove will help you stay on purpose.

6. Take time to visualize as well. Like speaking out loud, this carves new grooves and your subconscious goes to work to make it happen. Five minutes a day will speed up your progress.

7. Exercise. When it comes to exercise, think movement. If you aren't already active, getting started doesn't need to be elaborate or intense. It should be consistent. Know what you want to accomplish with movement: strength, core balance, build muscle, burn fat. You don't need to join a gym unless you want to. Do activities that are appropriate for your current level of health.

8. Keep a journal. If you use my *Diabetes Journal* you can track what you eat, your numbers, pictures of before and after, recipes that work for you, and journal how you are feeling, what trips you up and what brings the most success. The tracking is for a complete year, so you can either continue to track for a year or have room for stopping and picking back up again later. Whatever journal or food tracker you use, just don't skip this step.

9. Celebrate! It's important to celebrate your successes, however small. If you've messed up and gotten back on track, celebrate that! Give yourself rewards. Write down your milestones. You deserve it!

10. Connect with me at *Marian@MarianHays.com* if you have questions or need support. Every email will be answered.

22

Go For It!

Years ago, my husband and I went skiing for the first time in Durango, CO. At the top of the ski lift, he would ski down the blue slope while I took the green beginner run. Yes, the bunny slope. I never fell, not once. I was careful, a bit slow, but I didn't fall. Mike fell a few times, got up and kept going.

Next day I got brave and adventurous. No more green slope. If I fell, I fell. Without saying anything, we got off the ski lift. He took off down the blue slope, expecting me to repeat the bunny run.

When he glanced back, he saw me right behind him. I was following as closely as possible (and faster than I'd prefer) but I was determined to keep up. I only fell once or twice. I didn't break anything, and the blue run was great fun!

With only a day's experience of skiing and falling and getting back up, Mike became my coach, and I became a better skier. We had a blast!

My takeaway from this?

Something I remind myself from time to time. Break out! Never settle for past successes (like not falling on the safe slope). Take that next challenge. Set your bar higher.

Go farther. Do what others think can't be done. Amaze people. Amaze yourself!

We don't need to know everything to enjoy doing. And to make progress. We only get more information or see the next section of the map as we make progress with what information we have been given. Now it's your turn. I hope you're embracing that now.

You can amaze yourself as I did in stepping out with something new.

Life is a journey, not a destination. The most important step is the decision to make changes, however small. You've been through life experiences, good and bad, and made it to today. Now you can aim for a better, higher destination.

It's never a straight line to the top, but by making small corrections along the way, you can have a smoother ride from now on.

Be consistent and realize that it won't be an overnight one-time solution. You'll soon get into a rhythm of healthy choices. After a while, sweet or salty foods will no longer appeal to you the way they have in the past.

Dessert on a special occasion when you've been eating well shouldn't be a problem. You might backslide now and then, but you'll know how to get back on track.

Be sure to choose someone to work with and to hold you accountable in an encouraging way. A family member or close friend works well, especially if it's someone who is also on the same journey you are on. A coach is another great option.

I hope you choose a great lifestyle instead of a life sentence! You're worth it!

Here's to your great success in overcoming diabetes!

About the Author

Marian Hays writes, coaches, and speaks about health and empowering personal growth.

She's not an M.D. or a professional nutritionist, but an advocate for others as she researches and shares truth instead of hype.

Her group coaching program builds community as she guides and encourages others to stay on track to accomplish their objectives. She helps them identify strengths, uncover blocks, and learn ways to overcome them. They gain self-awareness to maximize their influence in personal, family and career success.

Marian and her husband live in Frisco, Texas.

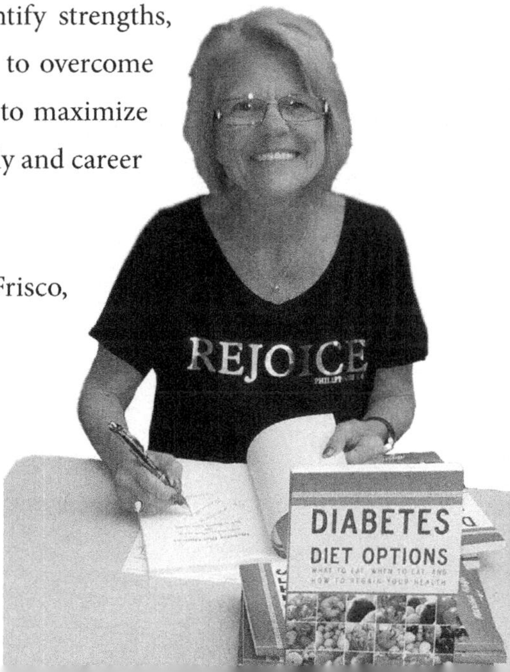

How to Work with Marian

Speaking: Bring Marian to your special interest group, book clubs, writing groups

Coaching/Training: Individual and group coaching is available. Join her group coaching or membership site for ongoing new ideas and information.

Books: Find her books at Amazon and other book retailers. If they're out of stock, ask for it by name. They can order it for you. We welcome your reviews.

Website: Check her websites for books and reports that will provide ongoing information about health and self-help such as mindset and other empowerment topics.

Email: Marian@MarianHays.com

Website: www.MarianHays.com

Blog: www.HealthAndEmpowerment.com

HealthAndEmpowerment-1911204955864743/

www.linkedin.com/in/mhays/

bit.do/MHaysYouTube

References

Diabetes Diet Options http://amzn.to/2vciTqU

Diabetes Journal http://amzn.to/2FYRj39

Web links

https://www.healthline.com/nutrition/fix-the-hormones-that-make-you-fat

https://www.lifetime-weightloss.com/blog/2012/6/2/insulin-and-fat-storage.html

https://www.medicalnewstoday.com/articles/318472.php

https://www.cdc.gov/media/releases/2017/p0718-diabetes-report.html

https://www.scientificamerican.com/article/gut-feelings-the-second-brain-in-our-gastrointestinal-systems-excerpt/

https://www.deathtodiabetes.com/diabetes-medications.php

http://www.sugar.ca/english/consumers/typessugar.cfm

http://www.sugar.ca/Nutrition-Information-Service/Consumers/About-Sugar/Types-of-Sugar.aspx

https://www.nlm.nih.gov

https://www.fda.gov

https://www.webmd.com/diabetes/news/20181221/2-types-of-diabetes-meds-may-raise-heart-risk#1

http://diabetes.niddk.nih.gov/

These websites monitor recalls, lawsuits and alerts:

http://www.fda.gov/drugs

https://www.drugwatch.com

http://www.recalls.gov/medicine.html_

http://www.drugrecallattorneysblog.com

http://rxrecall.com/drugs-a-z/

https://en.wikipedia.org/wiki/List_of_withdrawn_drugs

Books and Publications

Blood Sugar Solution 10-Day Detox Diet, Mark Hyman

Brain Warrior's Way, Dr. Daniel Amen

Change Your Brain Change Your Age, Dr. Daniel Amen

Change Your Brain Change Your Life, Dr. Daniel Amen

Daniel Plan, Rick Warren, Dr. Daniel Amen, Dr. Mark Hyman

Dr. Gundry's Diet Evolution, Dr. Steven Gundry

Food, Dr. Mark Hyman

Knowing-Doing Gap, Jeffrey Pfeiffer & Robert I. Sutton

Mindset, Carol S. Dweck, Ph.D.

Power of Habits, Charles Duhigg

Psycho-Cybernetics, Maxwell Maltz, MD, FICS

Resistance, Price Pritchett

TED Talk: Reversing Type 2 Diabetes Starts with Ignoring the Guidelines, Dr. Sarah Hallberg

Salt, Sugar, Fat, Michael Moss

Self-Disciplined Dieter, Martin Meadows

Sleep Smarter, Shawn Stevenson

Soul Detox, Craig Groeschel

Sugar and the Evil Empire, Geoff and Vicky Wells

Switch On Your Brain, Dr. Caroline Leaf

Triggers, Marshall Goldsmith

Walking in Divine Health, Don Colbert, M.D.

What Got You Here Won't Get You There, Marshall Goldsmith

What's Holding You Back? Linda Austin, M.D.

Willpower, Roy F. Baumeister and John Tierney

Your Body's Internal Clock and How It Affects Your Overall Health, Alice G. Walton, The Atlantic.com

Your Brain at Work, David Rock

Index

Your Reviews

If you found this book to be helpful, please leave a review at Amazon. You'll help others decide if this is a book for them, and the author will be very grateful. *Thanks!*

Made in the USA
Monee, IL
04 November 2026

67378968R00105